Aging in Good Health

A Quality Lifestyle for the Later Years

Aging in Good Health

A Quality Lifestyle for the Later Years

Edited by

Florence Lieberman, D.S.W.

and

Morris F. Collen, M.D.

INSIGHT BOOKS

PLENUM PRESS • NEW YORK AND LONDON

Library of Congress Cataloging in Publication Data

Lieberman, Florence.
Aging in good health: a quality lifestyle for the later years / edited by Florence Lieberman and Morris F. Collen.
p. cm.
Includes bibliographical references and index.
ISBN 0-306-44502-6
1. Aged—Medical care. I. Collen, Morris F. (Morris Frank), 1913– . II. Title.
[DNLM: 1. Health Services for the Aged. 2. Life Style—in old age. 3. Quality of Life. WT 30 L716a 1993]
RC952.L54 1993
362.1'9897—dc20
DNLM/DLC 93-28126
for Library of Congress CIP

ISBN 0-306-44502-6

A Division of Plenum Publishing Corporation
233 Spring Street, New York, N.Y. 10013

An Insight Book

Printed in the United States of America

To the memory of

STANLEY LESSE, M.D. (1922–1990)

A Founder and Chair of The National Academy of Practice in Medicine; Member of The Forum Program Committee; Editor, *American Journal of Psychotherapy*

Contributors

BARBARA BERKMAN, D.S.W., Director of Research and Quality Assurance, Social Service Department, Massachusetts General Hospital, Boston, Massachusetts

CHARLES R. BRANTINGHAM, D.P.M., Assistant Clinical Professor of Medicine, University of Southern California School of Medicine, Los Angeles, California

LEO K. BUSTAD, D.V.M., Ph.D., Professor and Dean Emeritus, Washington State University, and Director, People–Pet Partnership Program, Pullman, Washington

MORRIS F. COLLEN, M.D., Director Emeritus, Division of Research, Kaiser Permanente Medical Care Program, Oakland, California

NICHOLAS A. CUMMINGS, Ph.D., Litt.D., President, National Academies of Practice, and Founder and Chairman, American Biodyne, Inc., South San Francisco, California

WILLIAM R. FELTS, M.D., Professor of Medicine, George Washington University School of Medicine, Washington, D.C.

ALLAN N. FREID, O.D., F.A.A.O., Southern California College of Optometry, Fullerton, California

ARTHUR E. HELFAND, D.P.M., Professor and Chairman, Department of Community Health and Aging, Pennsylvania College of Podiatric Medicine, Philadelphia, Pennsylvania

SAUL KAMEN, D.D.S., F.A.C.D., Chief Emeritus of Dental Service, Parker Jewish Geriatric Institute, New Hyde Park, New York

ROSALIE A. KANE, D.S.W., Professor, School of Social Work and School of Public Health, University of Minnesota, Minneapolis, Minnesota

THOMAS LANGFITT, M.D., President, Pew Charitable Trust, Washington, D.C.

ARNOLD M. LEVIN, Ph.D., B.C.D., L.C.S.W., President, Institute for Clinical Social Work, Chicago, Illinois

FLORENCE LIEBERMAN, D.S.W., B.C.D., Chair, National Health Forum Committee, and Professor Emerita, Hunter College School of Social Work, City University of New York, New York, New York

WILLIAM M. LUDLAM, O.D., F.A.A.O., College of Optometry, Pacific University, Forest Grove, Oregon

ARNOLD M. LUDWIG, M.D., E. A. Edwards Professor of Psychiatry, University of Kentucky College of Medicine, Lexington, Kentucky

SANDRA MACKAY, R.N., Ph.D., School of Nursing, San Francisco State University, San Francisco, California

RICHARD MAYEUX, M.D., Professor of Neurology and Psychology, College of Physicians and Surgeons, Columbia University, New York, New York

LINDA R. PHILLIPS, Ph.D., R.N., Professor, College of Nursing, University of Arizona, Tucson, Arizona

BARBARA SILVERSTONE, D.S.W., Executive Director, The Lighthouse, New York, New York

WILLIAM SPENCER, M.D., Emeritus Professor of Rehabilitation Medicine, Baylor College of Medicine, Houston, Texas

GARY R. VANDENBOS, Ph.D., Executive Director, Office of Publications and Communications, American Psychological Association, Washington, D.C.

THELMA J. WELLS, R.N., Ph.D., F.A.A.N., F.R.C.N., Professor, School of Nursing, University of Rochester, Rochester, New York

Acknowledgments

The publication of this book would not have been possible without the help and encouragement of many people.

Norma Fox, Executive Editor, and Frank K. Darmstadt, Editor, Insight Books, suggested this informal presentation of the deliberations of the National Academies of Practice Health Forum on Problems of the Aging.

Terry Pickett patiently helped the various distinguished health practitioners, contributors to this book, rewrite their technical papers so that the language is more colloquial.

Many participants, distinguished practitioners of the National Academies of Practice, provided thoughtful comments about the health needs of the elderly. Beverly Carlson, Executive Secretary, facilitated communication between the editors and the various authors.

The editors thank all for their support.

Contents

Better Health Care for the Elderly

Introduction to an Interdisciplinary Approach

MORRIS F. COLLEN, M.D.

Many more people in the United States are now living longer, and their healthier young and middle years compress their morbidity into their later years of life. It is obvious that, if you escape all the other vicissitudes of life, the diseases of aging will get you in the end. One can safely predict that a thorough health checkup will find some significant variations from normality in everyone over sixty-five years old. Yet, some of the diseases of the elderly are preventable, and many are postponable. It is a harsh reality that, compared with younger age groups, the elderly have significantly more diseases that require more diagnostic and therapeutic procedures, they use more office visits to a greater variety of specialists, they spend more days in hospitals, they take many more medications, and their health care costs more. When the elderly are sick, they often suffer from a combination of abnormalities in different organ systems and body parts, they have diminished immune responses to stresses and slower recuperative capabilities, and their appropriate treatment often requires a multispecialty team of health professionals. The seriousness of this challenging problem can readily be demonstrated by such statistics as that almost half of all people eighty-five or older suffer from rheumatism, mental disorders, and/or impaired vision and hearing.

The elderly are especially vulnerable and fragile because any illness can adversely affect not only their physiological status, but also their psychological, social, and economic status. Most elderly people have multiple functional disabilities, the most common being impaired mobility. Treating the immediate medical problem that brings the patient to the health professional does not often cure such disabilities as impaired mobility, and treating such disabilities does not often cure the medical problem.

It has been estimated that by 1995, 13 percent of the total population of the United States will be sixty-five or older. The proportion of the elderly in our nation's population has reached such continually increasing levels that providing them appropriate, effective, accessible, and affordable care has become a high-priority national policy issue. Almost half of the annual United States medical expenditure goes to caring for persons in their last year of life, so the treatment of these patients has become a prime target for cost containment and the rationing of expensive care. Congress supports the care of the elderly through the provisions of the Medicare Act, and the Health Care Financing Agency (HCFA) partially reimburses hospitals and health professionals for their care of the elderly. Increasing health care costs have resulted in demands for a better assessment of the cost-effectiveness of diagnostic and therapeutic procedures, and for improved measures of the outcomes of patient care. Yet, such measures are difficult to apply to the elderly, as outcome implies the assessment of physical, mental, and psychosocial functioning. The quality of life in the elderly changes very rapidly with time and with the aging process itself, and a worsening in their general health often occurs despite adequate levels of care.

Reimbursement for the costs of preventive care for the elderly should be an important consideration because, for example: giving pneumococcal vaccine is cheaper than treating pneumonia; providing mammograms is cheaper than treating breast cancer, and 50 percent of breast cancers occur in women sixty-five or older; the prescription of an appropriate orthotic device for an arthritic foot may prevent immobility; and an appropriately fitted shoe costs less than a joint replacement.

The National Academies of Practice (NAP) addressed the complex and difficult problems associated with providing health care to the elderly by bringing together in a national forum an interdisciplinary group of recognized experts from each of its nine academies to share experiences and provide their respective insights into prevention, intervention, and care of the elderly. The NAP was founded in 1981 and is limited to 100 "Distinguished Practitioners" in each of the nine major health professions recognized by the Congress of the United States: dentistry, medicine, nursing, optometry, osteopathic medicine, podiatric medicine, psychology, social work, and veterinary medicine. The National Academies of Practice is unique in its commitment to interdisciplinary communication that will provide a balanced view of patient care; each national health-care issue is addressed by licensed practitioners in each of the nine major health professions. Thus, the experiences of all of these groups of practitioners are shared in the interests of improving the overall health care.

Each health practitioner cares for each patient as a whole, yet each focuses particularly on the abnormalities that he or she is licensed to treat. Although a basic geriatric assessment of an elderly patient can be performed by practitioners of any of the health care professions, this basic health-status evaluation must be augmented by the specialty assessments of each discipline. Physicians have the broadest responsibilities and have developed a specialty in geriatrics to coordinate their care of the illnesses of the elderly. The commonest of these conditions are heart disease, hypertension, arthritis, cancer, diabetes, cataracts, varicose veins, strokes, mental disorders, limited mobility, incontinence, adverse reactions to medications, and injuries. Unfortunately, many of the elderly suffer from several of these conditions at once.

Most elderly patients seen by physicians visit their medical offices, some patients are seen by their physicians in hospitals, and some are seen in their own homes or in nursing homes. Physicians who provide care for the elderly are increasingly affected by changing Medicare regulations. Physicians who care for aged patients often face ethical issues in the appropriate use of costly technology such as organ transplants, replacement joints, the use of intensive-care units for irreversible conditions, and the long-term use of life support systems. Health professionals urge that national policymakers' current emphasis on costs and on the effectiveness of health care delivery be appropriately balanced by the individual practitioner's obligations to satisfy each patient's and family's needs and expectations.

The major mental health problems among the elderly are dementia and severe cognitive impairment, depression and other mood disorders, suicide, the misuse of alcohol and drugs, and the improper use of over-the-counter and prescription medications. A major challenge to psychiatrists and psychologists is to meet the special needs of older people who have impaired cognitive abilities, increased levels of stress, and problems in obtaining adequate mental health care. Illness in the elderly often results in debility, depression, dependency, and disengagement. Psychologists find that many of the common emotional and behavioral problems of the elderly are treatable, and that elderly patients often do benefit from psychotherapy. Yet, many of the mental health needs of the elderly are not met. Psychologists advocate further changes in the policies governing their practice to facilitate access to, and to expand the range of, their services to the elderly.

The majority of all direct patient care of the elderly is provided by nurses. Nurses implement the care plans for patients in hospitals, and the nursing profession has the major role in the care of the elderly in home care and nursing-home care. Although a long-term illness often does not require a stay in an acute-care hospital, some level of nursing care underlies all care of the elderly, either in nursing homes or in the patients' homes by visiting home nurses or by nurse extenders (nursing assistants or family caregivers). Nurses define their role in the care of elderly patients as the management of clinical problems, the prevention of functional decline, and the promotion of health.

Gerontological nursing practitioners advocate a more proactive national policy of preventing disease and disability that will educate people to adopt more healthy lifestyles and will foster innovative living arrangements for the elderly as alternatives to nursing homes.

The dental professional emphasizes that oral disease in the elderly differs from that in younger persons, and that oral diseases influence the management of elderly patients who also have other diseases. Geriatric dental practitioners urge all health professionals to support national policies and programs that will provide the elderly easier access to and improved practices for the treatment and prevention of their dental disorders.

Optometrists cite the statistic that two-thirds of the visually impaired in the United States are over age sixty-five. The conditions that most commonly cause this impairment of vision are cataracts, retinal conditions resulting from systemic conditions (e.g., hypertension, diabetes, and nephritis), and retinal conditions resulting from ocular abnormalities (e.g., glaucoma, retinal detachment, and macular degeneration). Optometry, in cooperation with ophthalmology, urges better service for the elderly to meet what optometrists state is one of the largest unmet health care needs in this country: adequate vision care.

Practitioners of podiatric medicine remind us that healthy feet are important to general health, and that the ability of the elderly to walk is critical to their maintaining their independence. Thus, good foot care is very important to the elderly. For elderly patients with diabetes, foot care assumes an additional importance in the prevention of infection and gangrene. The treatment of diabetic foot conditions, which traditionally has involved a variety of health professions, serves as a model of the interdisciplinary approach to important health problems of the elderly. Podiatrists emphasize that adequate and timely assessment and care of the feet can prevent many foot impairments in the elderly. They advocate education of all health professionals and caregivers in the essentials of foot health in their elderly patients.

Social workers have been increasingly involved in the interaction of psychosocial processes and illnesses in the elderly. They are frequently called on to assist elderly hospitalized patients and their families to clarify the alternatives available to the patients on leaving the hospital. For approximately half of all elderly patients, social workers provide discharge planning for posthospital care services. When planning their patients' long-term care needs, they often confront such psychological factors as anxiety, depression, and denial in elderly patients who are leaving the hospital. Social workers develop discharge plans for the elderly patients in nursing homes and provide the bridge between the nursing home or extended-care facility and the family caregiver and the community. They consider the social support (advice, guidance, material aid, and services) available from family, friends, and community resources. As case managers and care coordinators for those elderly who require long-term care for chronic disease or disability, social workers provide guidance in the appropriate use of a comprehensive variety of community-based care services. Forty percent of patients over eighty-five use long-term care for their chronic problems, and in such cases, all health-care disciplines are involved. Surveys of the elderly have indicated that they place a very high importance on maintaining their independence, ambulation, vision, and nutrition.

Practitioners of veterinary medicine emphasize the beneficial effects of the interaction of the elderly with animals. They cite many animal interaction programs for elderly people who are disabled or institutionalized, programs that have been reported to improve patients' alertness, increase their morale, lower their depression, and reduce their demands for care. The veterinary profession advocates working together with other health professionals to increase the "human–animal bond" so as to improve the health of the elderly and also the well-being of the animals involved.

In the remainder of the 1990s, it is hoped that innovations in technology will permit more care of the elderly to move out of the hospital and into the office and the home. Personal computers in the home with modems connected to telephone lines will permit practice-linked clinical support and education of the family to upgrade the quality of home care. The advent of portable computer-based patient records will improve the continuity of care given to a patient at different sites. Health care policy, it is hoped, will help support home caregivers and increase the funding for prevention and rehabilitation. Meeting all of the stiff challenges in improving the care of the elderly in our country is not possible for any one group of health care practitioners. The National Academies of Practice brings together the different health professions so that, rather than compete with each other for the care of the elderly, they cooperate in best satisfying the needs of these patients. The NAP seeks to bring about this collaboration, and to apply the combined experience and wisdom of all the appropriate health-care disciplines to this high-priority problem.

I

HEALTH CARE FOR BETTER LIVING

1

Cost-Effective Health Care of the Elderly

An Internist's Perspective

WILLIAM R. FELTS, M.D.

It is impossible to divorce the internist's services to an individual patient from the complex socioeconomic cauldron that constitutes the American health-care system. Accordingly, it is appropriate to review a number of items that are currently affecting medical practice. It is hoped that ongoing discussions to revise present health practices will address the issues that are of importance to both patients and the providers of health services.

Practice Environment

Among the challenges in the practice environment are (1) an aging population with a burden of increasing comorbidities (the occurrence of two or more diseases at the same time); (2) an explosion of expensive diagnostic and therapeutic technologies; (3) geographically scattered technical resources; (4) a plethora of expensive pharmaceuticals; (5) inordinate demands for information by third parties; (6) inadequate reimbursement for cognitive and case-management skills as compared with procedure performance; (7) increasing Medicare requirements of data and codes that meet detailed criteria; (8) encouragement by hospitals to discharge ill patients unless they meet a guideline of need for acute care, as well as challenges by peer review organizations (PROs) when this guideline is not met; (9) pressures from patients for assistance in bypassing deductible and coinsurance requirements; and (10) a progressively more litigious climate.

Answering requests for counseling, listening to concerns outside those necessary for diagnosis and prescribing, and responses to telephone queries impose unscheduled demands that are largely not paid for. The requirements of attending and actively participating in hospital rounds, conferences, continuing medical education, and the committee activities of institutions in order to maintain admitting privileges add to the unreimbursed intrusions on the physician's time. These irritants disturb the flow of professional practice and impinge upon the most important task which is attending to the patient's health needs.

Attributes of the Elderly

Some of the characteristics of the aged further expand the time required for their care, for example, their longer medical histories and the frequent presence of comorbid conditions with a myriad of symptoms affecting several body systems. It is not unusual, especially when the patient is one of the "older elderly," to need a family member in attendance to confirm and amplify the historical details. Many elderly require greater assistance in preparing for their examinations, as well as repetitive explanations of abnormal findings, prescriptions, and other instructions.

Social and medical problems are often intermingled and sometimes inseparable. The need for guidance into the purview of social and home-health-care agencies; repetitive consulting with the agency; the establishment of appropriate referrals to specialists or geographically more accessible physicians; the acquisition and compilation of old records to minimize redundant and expensive retesting; and the assurance that appropriate follow-up will occur—all add to the internist's services. Patients seeing multiple physicians require vigilance against the risks of polypharmacy and drug interactions. Patient compliance in following medical regimens, abetted by "forgetfulness," is uncertain. As patients grow older, senile dementias may also create confusion in the physician's judging the patients' needs and demands.

The Aging Population

Our population is aging. In 1900, only 5 percent were sixty-five or older. By 1985, 12 percent of the U.S. resident population had reached this age, and by 2025, this proportion will reach 20 percent. Of this contingent, 1.1 percent are 85 and over, the most rapidly growing segment of the elderly. Between 1970 and 1984, life expectancy at age sixty-five increased by 1.0 to 1.7 years, depending on the race and sex of the subgroup; in the 1990s this growth is continuing.

This increase in the numbers of elderly is a tribute to the achievements of American medicine and research, and to the public health measures that contribute to longevity. The medical profession also dedicates itself to supporting the patient's desire to enjoy independent living, to maximize self-care, and to attain the highest quality of life possible within her or his limitations.

Medicare

Alfred, Lord Tennyson, wrote:

> Forward, forward let us range,
> Let the great world spin forever
> down the ringing grooves of change.

The Medicare program for the elderly is involved in seemingly endless "grooves of change." Its initial enactment in 1965 acknowledged the pluralistic nature of American health care. It provided statutory recognition of regional differences, the patient's freedom to choose a provider, the separation of hospital expenses (Part A) from ambulatory care and physician services (Part B), and usual and customary fee reimbursement. It also reassured the medical profession that the law would "not be used to change medical practice."

However, almost all "top-down" regulatory systems eventually result in inequities for some individuals. Regulatory and statutory patchwork efforts made in subsequent years have attempted to repair and strengthen the program. Nonetheless, the third-party mechanisms have stimulated many of the current problems, and the practice of medicine *has* changed. I will later discuss both of these topics in more depth.

Unresolved Societal Issues

The question of "Health Care as a Right" is an unsettled societal issue that continues to affect considerations in expanding health care benefits. From a strictly legal perspective, neither the U.S. Supreme Court nor any appellate court has found a constitutional right to health or health care. The need for universal health care is obvious. Yet no discussion of "rights" can ignore the issue of adequate provision for their "costs."

Former Governor Scott Matheson of Utah observed:

> It is interesting to note that there are millions of Americans who are homeless, yet society does not require home builders and contractors to provide homes for them free of charge or at prices below the costs of construction. Millions of Americans go to bed hungry every night, yet society does not require farmers or grocery store chains to feed them free of charge or at substantially discounted prices . . . but . . . society at times appears to believe that health providers . . . should provide care free, or at the least cost, for those who cannot afford it.[1]

The President's Commission for the Study of Ethical Problems in Medicine concluded in 1983 that, instead of speaking in terms of "rights," recommendations are better expressed in terms of "ethical and moral obligation."

Stanley B. Jones, a consultant on the financing of health care services, can be paraphrased in his perceptions of the business community:

> It is not clear that we [Americans] *really* want to provide expanded access to health care. Employers are worried about their labor markets, the rising costs of doing business, and competitiveness in the world market. In the fast-growing services industries, employers find it is not always necessary to provide health insurance coverage. Providers appear more comfortable with add-ons in technology and sophisticated procedures than in extending access to primary or preventive care. Insurers in the competitive environment are looking for profitable and self-supporting markets; not markets that are risky or economically marginal. Insured individuals want the best deal for their premiums . . . if benefits are to be extended, how are monies to be raised?[2]

Other, equally difficult societal questions have been posed, such as: Do the elderly have an obligation to step aside? Need physicians try to save *every* life, including the life of those who do not want to be saved? If resources are to be rationed, who is to do the rationing?

Shifting Medicare Emphasis

Karen Davis observed that, in the 1950s and 1960s, the nation's programmatic emphasis was on access to care. As access improved, costs expanded far beyond the actuarial levels originally envisioned, and the government's focus shifted toward cost control. In the 1990s, it is obvious that a third major factor is to be scrutinized: the effectiveness and quality of care.

Thinking about Costs

As we consider the challenge to provide cost-effective care, what are some issues that influence our thinking about increased costs?

Personal attitudes and the age of retirement are influential. Legislatively established caps have stimulated many to retire between sixty-five and seventy. The desire to continue working into the later years reflects a complex interplay among financial need and reward, gratification attained through work, and the functional capacity to meet job demands. Sixty percent of those who worked at some time following their sixty-fifth birthday can still perform work-related activities if they retire for reasons other than health, but only 14 percent can do so if they retire because of their health. More significantly, very few of these potential workers wanted to be employed. Therefore, whether the recent modifications of the retirement laws will result in a change of the age at which people retire means to be seen. Fixed income levels after retirement affect the attitudes of older Americans, as they have less flexibility in dealing with increased and unanticipated costs.

The shadow of the national debt is also influencing the American mind-set. At the end of the 1980s, the federal government finally began to acknowledge the fact that an overly indebted nation cannot survive indefinitely. It reluctantly began the arduous process of grappling with the reality that the nation's spending is transferring the national debt to our children and grandchildren in an intergenerational impact that is intolerable to most of us as individuals. Pragmatic reality interferes with our ethical and moral inclinations to provide necessary health care to all individuals.

Factors Affecting Costs

An explosion has occurred in technological development and new procedures. Magnetic resonance imaging (MRI) machines, which yield much greater soft-tissue detail than prior methods, were introduced in 1982. Organ transplants became clinically more commonplace, and even multiorgan transplants emerged in 1989. Laser surgery has become widely available, and genetic engineering has become a clinical reality. Life-sustaining equipment has become more effective and has stimulated greater costs and seemingly endless debates on new ethical issues. A new disease, AIDS, has become epidemic, has so far defied scientific solution, and is currently consuming many medical resources.

The technological explosion was accompanied by a change in patient expectations, and professional lawsuits proliferated as patients and attorneys focused on undesired outcomes in addition to actual malpractice. Unconscionable premiums for liability insurance resulted, and some physicians began to abandon the practice of high-risk procedures. Thus, the dilemma imposed by increased costs has continued to grow.

Medical Conditions Common to the Elderly

When we examine the reasons for the office visits of those fifty-five and older, the most common medical problems are essential hypertension, diabetes, chronic ischemic heart disease (in which the arterial blood flow to the heart is impaired), and osteoarthritis. All are diseases that generally require continuing rather than episodic medical care. Trends in the prevalence of these conditions increase among certain subgroups of persons fifty-five and older. Osteoarthritis is present in more than one-half of females aged sixty-five and older. Impairments in vision and hearing are more common in each consecutively older age group. Injury rates are higher after age eighty-five.

The economic cost and social impact of chronic illness in the United States can be illustrated by the rheumatic diseases. In 1980, the $21-billion expenditures for health care and for lost wages due to these conditions were equivalent to about 1 percent of the gross national product. These conditions also accounted for 5 percent of all hospitalizations, 10 percent of all hospital procedures, and 9 percent of all physician visits. Over two million persons were rendered incapable of performing major activities, five million were otherwise limited, and at least one million were severely impaired in their activities of daily living. This impact is likely to grow, because population aging increases both the prevalence and the severity of the rheumatic diseases. It is apparent that more intensive research on these common chronic illnesses is needed.

Comorbidity and Disability

The importance of comorbidities (the presence of two or more diseases) among the elderly and the need to address greater attention to them have also been revealed in statistical studies. National 1984 estimates of the prevalence of comorbid conditions in those over age sixty focused on eight common conditions: osteoarthritis (present in 49 percent of comorbidities); cataracts (19.9 percent); heart disease (14 percent); varicose veins (9.9 percent); diabetes (9.5 percent); cancer, exclusive of non-melanoma skin malignancies (6.6 percent); osteoporosis or hip fracture (5.5 percent); and stroke (5.4 percent). The number of comorbid conditions was higher at each older age and was higher in women than men. These conditions are still problems today.

Disability rises markedly in the presence of comorbidity and with increasing numbers of comorbid conditions. It also increases gradually with age. Hypertension and arthritis, the two conditions with the highest prevalence, co-occur in 24.1 percent of those sixty and older; cataract and arthritis, in 11.7 percent. Seven of the eight most common pairs of conditions demonstrate more comorbidity than expected. The prevalence of comorbidity for women rises from 45 percent in those sixty to sixty-nine to 70 percent in those eighty and older. These percentages of diagnoses of comorbidity appear to offer a useful measure of the burden of illness on the older individual and its associated disability.

Selected Demographics and Long-Term Care

Long-term-care needs require special attention. The "spend-down" requirement for families before they can achieve eligibility for Medicaid assistance has resulted in couples' using their marital assets for nursing-home care, so that many surviving spouses are impoverished during their remaining years. In 1985, less than 5 percent of the population aged sixty-five and older, 10 percent aged seventy-five and older, and 22 percent aged eighty-five and older resided in nursing homes, but these percentages are increasing.

About 26.4 million persons aged sixty-five and older live in communities outside nursing homes or other institutions. About one-third (8.4 million) live alone, and those living alone tend to be older, widowed, and female. Many living alone are *not* disabled, in poor health, suffering from the lack of medical care, or lacking family or other companionship.

Persons eighty-five and older constitute a disproportionate share of all persons dependent in their physical functioning, including home management, personal care, mobility activities, and daily incontinence.

Home care has been considered more desirable than institutional care, even though the definition of home care is extraordinarily vague. About 80 percent of home care is provided free by friends and relatives. But two Health Care Financing Administration (HCFA) research studies in Georgia and California, which evaluated the feasibility of substituting home and community services for nursing-home admissions, failed to confirm expectations. Some services had been presumed to be effective in preventing patients from requiring nursing-home admission. During the study, it was found that such was not the case; in both the control group and the services-provided group, the same number of people ended up in a nursing home. Therefore, "targeting" such services to specific patients would not be warranted on a cost-effectiveness basis. Some have concluded that home care in the future for the vast majority of the elderly is likely to be open-ended, to make little use of volunteer staff, and to serve a population that both is older and has more varied needs than in the past.

Enhancing Data

Recognition of the importance of more detailed data that will enable better planning of future health care for the elderly led in 1986 to the establishment of a Federal Interagency Forum on Aging-Related Statistics. Its purpose is to encourage cooperation among federal agencies in the development, collection, analysis, and dissemination of data pertaining to the older population. Additional efforts to improve national data include expanding the Third National Health and Nutrition Examination Survey (NHANES III) to incorporate persons aged seventy-five and older for the first time; expanding the National Health Care Survey to cover the major providers of care to older persons, including ambulatory surgical centers, home health agencies, and hospices; making a survey of the dynamics of aging to address the need for longitudinal data; and conducting cognitive interviews with the young-old (sixty-five to seventy) and the oldest-old (eighty and older) to test the adequacy of the existing survey questions to collect information from people with certain disabilities and functional limitations.

The Medicare Dilemma

Medicare's expansion via the enactment of the Catastrophic Health Act in 1988 failed to satisfy the concerns of the elderly, and there was a drop in satisfaction with the Medicare program, from 70 percent to 30 percent. The act was repealed the following year. A major cause of its rejection was the logical fiscal approach adopted by the Congress, which placed a significant premium burden for the expanded benefits on the potential users, the elderly themselves. The reaction of those on Medicare was somewhat of a paradox, as one survey indicated that more than 78 percent had purchased private insurance to supplement their Medicare coverage and thereby to minimize the deductible and coinsurance gaps.

Unfortunately, few appear to realize that the Medicare program is fiscally unsound and, barring significant changes, headed for bankruptcy. Some believe that the entire program needs to be restructured.

Although there are currently about four workers paying taxes to support each Medicare beneficiary, by the middle of the next century there will be only two workers for each beneficiary. According to the Medicare trustees, by the year 2005 the Medicare Part A trust fund will be totally exhausted. It could be $1 trillion in debt by the year 2010, according to recent estimates by former Department of Health and Human Services Secretary

Louis Sullivan. The Medicare financing system is pay-as-you-go, creates an intergenerational transfer of resources, and is adversely affected by the deteriorating worker-to-beneficiary ratio. It also lacks true catastrophic protection for acute care, lacks equitable means-testing (assessing a person's finances to determine eligibility for assistance) to help keep costs down, and requires increasingly burdensome government administration.

Medicare Programmatic Responses in the 1980s

As the major focus of government shifted from access to costs, a bewildering battery of legislative changes made the already-complicated Medicare rules almost indecipherable for patients and physicians alike. Some examples follow.

In 1983, diagnosis-related groups (DRGs) were imposed in an attempt to cap hospital expenditures. Further regulatory impositions included utilization review, preadmission approval requirements, and second opinions for surgery. Managed-care options through health maintenance organizations (HMOs), preferred-provider organizations (PPOs), and similar mechanisms were stimulated.

Congress also became more attentive to physician reimbursement. The geographic location and the economic fortunes of the region affect individual physician income, but the major determining factor has been specialty. Studies have confirmed the allegations by primary-care specialties that the charge-based method of payment has discriminated against them and favored specialists.

Congress has intervened to redistribute reimbursement among doctors and to curtail the growth of costs. A fee freeze was threatened in 1982, and mandatory assignment, or acceptance of the Medicare-determined reimbursement for service (usually considerably lower than the physician's usual charges), on inpatient claims was sought unsuccessfully by some in the Congress in 1983. In 1984, a fifteen-month fee freeze was enacted that dragged on for twenty-eight months. A significant disparity between assignment- and non-assignment-accepting physicians was created. The legislators pruned more than $10 billion from the Medicare program and enacted more than $4 billion in physician pay curbs. The Congress also established the Physician Payment Review Commission (PPRC).

In 1984, the HCFA was directed by statute to fund a study of a resource-based relative value scale (RBRVS) as a possible basis for a national fee schedule. This study determined a work value for each procedure or service performed by physicians. Also determined was the cost of providing services, practice overhead, and professional liability costs. The resulting "total relative work values," when multiplied by a dollar conversion factor (to be set by the Department of Health and Human Services or the Congress) has resulted in a national fee schedule for each service provided by physicians. All doctors in the Medicare program are paid on a fee-for-service basis according to this schedule.

The Congress enacted provisions to implement this RBRVS for physicians in the Medicare program as part of the Omnibus Budget Reconciliation Act of 1989 (OBRA 1989, P.L. 101–239) in the last hours before Thanksgiving adjournment. (It began to be phased in over five years beginning in 1992.) Among other provisions, it limits the extent to which government can cut fee growth in order to make up for Medicare expenditures that exceed those projected for the previous year.

To address the "effectiveness-of-care" issue, an OBRA statute mandated the establishment of an Agency for Health Care Policy and Research (AHCPR) under the aegis of the U.S. Public Health Service. A broad base of scientific research and promotion of improvements in clinical practice and in the organization of financing and the delivery of health care services are authorized. The program focuses on the effectiveness, efficiency, and quality of services; the outcomes of services and procedures; clinical practice; health care technologies, facilities, and equipment; health care costs, productivity, and market forces; health promotion and disease prevention; health statistics and epidemiology; and medical liability.

An Office of the Forum for Quality and Effectiveness in Health Care was established within the agency. It periodically reviews and updates the relevant clinical guidelines used in determining how diseases, disorders, and other health care conditions can most effectively and appropriately be prevented, diagnosed, treated, and managed. By January 1, 1991, at least three sets of guidelines had been completed for clinical treatments of conditions that account for a significant portion of Medicare expenditures and that show a meaningful variation in the frequency or types of treatment provided.

Several national medical specialty societies and the American Medical Association (AMA) have been developing practice parameters for a number of years. Some of them may serve as a nucleus for initial activity by the AHCPR. There is a danger that "cookbook medicine" will result if strict adherence to guidelines is required. Inflexible interpretations in the presence of symptoms or signs that may indicate comorbid conditions may interfere with adequate diagnostic investigations and may become disadvantageous to patients. Therefore, close cooperative efforts between organized medicine, government, insurers, and others will be necessary to ensure that patients will be properly protected.

These limited examples reflect the Medicare program's incremental approach to regulatory control.

Medicare Reform Proposals

A number of proposals for Medicare reform have emerged, besides those undertaken by the government.

The most ambitious effort to review the nation's health care was "The Health Policy Agenda for the American People." Stimulated and initiated by the American Medical Association in 1982, this group of over 425 representatives from 172 different health, health-related, business, government, and consumer groups met over a period of five years to examine current and future concerns confronting the health sector into the next century. The group functioned under the premise that a consensus approach among knowledgeable people would yield reasonable, workable results.

One hundred and fifty-nine principles were derived. Some of the provisions in OBRA 1989 reflect a number of them. The private insurance community has responded by increasing its offerings of long-term-care insurance. Some are modifying their life insurance programs to enable the insured to use accumulated funds to pay for catastrophic health care.

A second example is "A Proposal for Financing Health Care for the Elderly," developed by the AMA and endorsed by its House of Delegates in June 1986. H.R. 2600, introduced into the 101st Congress by Congressman Charles Rose of North Carolina, proposed this approach. The bill would have:

- Maintained access to affordable high-quality health care for the elderly.
- Provided for a prefunded program.
- Provided for comprehensive protection, including catastrophic coverage.
- Provided for equitable means testing.
- Provided benefits through the private sector in a variety of ways, allowing individuals the flexibility to select from private plans that would give the beneficiary a choice in the source of coverage.
- Allowed for additional contributions to and tax-advantaged withdrawals from individual retirement accounts (IRAs) for funding supplemental elderly health-care expenses.
- Provided for a gradual increase in the age of eligibility.

This type of program, by significantly reducing the tax burden, would have cost taxpayers, individuals, and employers substantially less than maintaining the current Medicare program over the long run. It was devised to place the program on a sound fiscal basis, to eliminate the intergenerational transfer of debt, and to stimulate a greater sense of responsibility and participation on the part of individual beneficiaries.

A third recent suggestion for addressing the costs of health care in America asserts:

> We must set national priorities. In short, we must ration health care, starting with the simplest, most easily accomplished methods; at the same time seeking more informa-

> tion from the growing field of health services research. . . . Certainly, setting national standards and priorities should lead to a more rational allocation of our nation's resources.[3]

Caution should be the watchword in addressing formal rationing. National health systems in foreign nations have resulted in substantial losses by patients of freedom of choice and access to the fruits of research. Varying degrees of implicit and explicit rationing of care exist in most of them, imposed by the techniques of queuing, or taking one's turn for services; withheld technology; and triage, or prioritizing the treatment of patients according to the seriousness of the condition. Most Americans appear unaware of these implications and may not recognize them at all until it is too late. These issues and others are presently the focus of discussion by President Clinton's task force and by Congress.

Coping by an Internist

These "grooves of change" confirm that many current practice problems are beyond the scope of solution by the individual internist. It has become frustratingly difficult to provide high-quality, cost-effective care. Two major pathways by which to cope exist: through medical organizations and as an individual.

Participation in organizations may be passive (paying dues) or active (getting involved). Many organizational opportunities exist via umbrella groups such as the AMA or state or county medical associations; within specialty societies, such as the American Society of Internal Medicine (ASIM) or the American College of Physicians (ACP); via subspecialty groups; or through active service on a hospital medical staff. All are important.

A timely example, relevant to internists, of the effectiveness of such activities is the resource-based relative value scale (RBRVS). Over a decade ago, the ASIM popularized the phrase *cognitive services,* which involves decision making of varying degrees of complexity and the formulation of therapeutic (management) programs for the patient. Stepwise, the ASIM developed background materials, definitions, and proposals. A slowly progressive groundswell of recognition of the problem by the public and the Congress resulted. The ACP, the AMA, and the American Academy of Family Practice (AAFP) also became supportive of the concept. The eventual result was the enactment of the statutory framework in OBRA 1989 for reforming physician payment under Medicare via the RBRVS. Although the final chapter remains to be written on the success of this approach, primary-care physicians expected to be more fairly compensated for their services to the elderly following its implementation, which also could alleviate a number of the previously identified problems.

Of the many unresolved issues confronting physicians, the need for tort reform pertaining to professional liability probably heads the list. Research has shown that most claims are made and paid not on the basis of malpractice, but because of an undesired outcome caused by no acts of malpractice or negligence. These claims contribute greatly, both directly and indirectly, to medical costs without increasing benefits. A change or changes in this system are perceived to be highly desirable—another problem highly dependent on public support for solution. This is an area where state rather than national activities have been most effective to date. One must hope that the will of Americans to maintain and sustain the world's best health-care system will prevail in further addressing this problem.

Although high-quality care is being provided, from these remarks it is apparent that the ability of the individual internist to continue to provide such care is threatened; indeed, the survival of the specialty is not a foregone conclusion. The strongest tool in the internist's armamentarium for the elderly remains "personalized care." The term implies a complete knowledge of the patient's medical problems over time and a reasonable awareness of the patient's socioeconomic limitations. This knowledge allows the internist to be attuned to new symptoms, or to amplifications of old ones, and thus to be alert to a possible need for further investigations. Individualization of medications within the patient's tolerance is also desirable, as some older patients attain the desired result with lower doses of drugs than average and experience toxic responses at normal therapeutic levels. The timely and compatible selection of necessary consultants is also made easier.

When longitudinal care exists, a bond of trust usually develops between the patient and the internist that enhances health management and patient satisfaction. Fears of lawsuits, which may result in excessive diagnostic interventions so as "not to miss anything," when intuitive judgment dictates guarded restraint to be more appropriate, are less frequent.

A reprogramming of some current behavior may be necessary. For example, most internists were taught to freely utilize diagnostic procedures; it was a "sin" to make rounds with the professor and to be unable to demonstrate that Diagnoses X, Y, and Z had been ruled out. But with time, the process of elimination has become much more expensive, and the statistical likelihood of rare conditions contributing to the problem is often low. Older patients, their comorbidities, and their frailties are especially vulnerable to overtesting, and to complications brought on by the treatment itself. The idea that "more care means better care" must be challenged. Many tests and procedures can be repeated at less frequent intervals; greater reliance on clinical judgment should evolve. Patients will need to evidence a willingness to participate in these changes.

Office Business Procedures

The internist's office practice environment also requires fine-tuning. Dealing efficiently with the ever-increasing paperwork is a must. One method is the development of individual practice-encounter forms with precoded services, procedures, diagnoses, symptoms, and other reasons for encounters. The stringent, specific guidelines for diagnosis coding in ambulatory settings under Medicare will be increasingly enforced. A front-end investment of time by the internist to familiarize herself or himself with details, and to extract those descriptors and codes from the ninth revision of the International Classification of Diseases, Clinical Modification (ICD-9-CM), that most commonly describe the attributes of her or his patients will obviate spending more time and effort later.

Computerized billing, claims form completions (mandated for all physicians of all Medicare patients after September 1, 1990), and detailed itemizations of specific services, payments, and balances also expedite function. Electronic billing is growing in popularity and use and generally shortens the turnaround time for payment, thereby improving cash flow. Computer-generated appointment reminders reduce the problem of no-shows, to which some elderly are especially prone.

The maintenance of laboratory data flowsheets assists in following trends in the patient and provides a quick source of comprehensive information to the referring and consulting physicians and to hospital house staff when the patient requires hospitalization. Chronological medical-event summary-sheets that delineate the patient's major problems over time facilitate the recall of events and the discovery of their possible interrelationships. Computerized medical records may also be a wave of the future. Some of these approaches involve time trade-offs, but they contribute to efficiency and the quality of the care provided.

The internist must stay informed about regulatory requirements. The expanding world of universal provider identification numbers (UPINs), mandatory diagnostic codes, and possibly even Karnovsky codes of patient functional assessment to be assigned at each encounter displays no signs of abating. The ICD-10 (10th revision) will be implemented in the Medicare program. Its coding will change to alphanumeric and will require significant modifications of office forms and computer software. Timely anticipation will minimize work disruption.

Conclusion

The internist must continue his or her struggle for the immediate future to provide cost-effective health care. Partial relief may be on the way following a full implementation of the RBRVS.

A current approach to Medicare reform appears to be based

on the assumption that an evaluation of the outcome of the various interventions used in the management of specific diseases will eliminate those proven less effective or ineffective and will result in sufficient savings to sustain and expand medical care. It is a laudable goal.

However, there are no guarantees of the success of this approach. Some of the technical components needed to support the approach now exist. Methodologies are emerging for enhanced health services research. Better methods of gathering and utilizing national data are in operation. But the magnitude of the economic need is great, and the ability of the current financing methods to sustain the Medicare program remains suspect. The development of other options short of a national health service must continue to be encouraged and explored.

Notes

1. Scott Matheson, The Richard and Hinda Rosenthal Lectures, "Providing Universal and Affordable Health Care," Institute of Medicine, National Academy of Sciences, Washington, DC, 1989.
2. Stanley B. Jones, The Richard and Hinda Rosenthal Lectures, "Providing Universal and Affordable Health Care," Institute of Medicine, National Academy of Sciences, Washington, DC, 1989.
3. N. F. Davies and L. H. Felder, "Applying Brakes to the Runaway American Health Care System," *Journal of the American Medical Association* 263:1 (1989), pp. 73–76.

Suggested Reading

The Richard and Hinda Rosenthal Lectures, "Providing Universal and Affordable Health Care," Institute of Medicine, National Academy of Sciences, Washington, DC, 1989.

W. R. Felts, "Medicare and Physician Reimbursement—A Rational Viewpoint: The AMA Perspective," *Bulletin of New York Academy of Medicine* 64:1 (1988), pp. 75–89.

The Health Policy Agenda for the American People, ISBN 0-89970-2305; Summary Report, ISBN 0-89970-7; Reference Report, ISBN 0-89970-230-9, 1987.

2

The Physician's Role in the Rehabilitation of the Elderly

WILLIAM SPENCER, M.D.

Introduction

Restorative medicine and comprehensive rehabilitation emphasize prevention and early control of disability at any age. This emphasis is significantly different from many of the attitudes, expectations, management, and use of resources of those providing typical acute and chronic care. The role of the physician in the control of a disability derives from more than biological causes because other interactive factors, both personal and environmental, are equally important. These include the identification of the patient's potential to benefit from treatment and simultaneous personal management, as well as the arrangement of allied professional services and technical support. The latter are required to control the effects of changing adaptive personal physiological and psychological conditions and the restoration of functional capacities within the context of the location of daily life activities.

The disabled person, in conjunction with many professional and technical persons, may be involved in achieving effective performance in the activities of daily living that may overcome the social handicaps and environmental barriers associated with the aura of disability. The particular concerns of the older person, which may differ from those of the younger person, affect the timing and the scope of the total rehabilitative process. Early anticipatory management of disability is the unifying and crucial feature of the physician's role. A cardinal activity is the recognition and preservation of the personhood of those seeking help and guidance.

Impairment, Disability, and Handicap

Understanding the distinction between impairment, disability, and handicap is crucial to the process of restorative medicine and comprehensive rehabilitation.

Impairment was initially defined as a cause of functional limitation, and *disability* was defined as a decrease in independence, mobility, leisure activities, social integration, and economic viability (individual consequences); a need for care, disturbed social relationships, and an economic burden (family consequences); and a demand for care, loss of productivity, and disturbed social integration (societal consequences).

More recently, *disability* has come to be considered the same as *functional limitation,* and the concept of *handicap* has been added. Currently, *impairment* is any loss or abnormality of a psychological, physiological, or anatomical structure or function, thus of the individual parts of the body; a *disability* is any restriction on or lack of ability to perform an activity in the manner or range considered normal, these activities including compound and integrated activities, tasks, skills, or behaviors; and a *handicap* is a disadvantage that limits or prevents the fulfillment of a role that is normal for that individual. Age, sex, social, and cultural factors and physical barriers are also considered. Thus, a handicap includes environmental factors impeding the functional restoration of participation in appropriate social activities of daily life.

These distinctions are important because the primary focus of medicine, social programs, and reimbursement is on discrete impairments or diseases. A straightforward cure or prevention is the exclusive purpose and emphasis of most research. A ready example of category restriction is found in the disease designations, such as arthritis or metabolic diseases, of fund-raising groups and even the National Institutes of Health. This position is ludicrous because disability is often a major consequence of many of these diseases.

I am convinced that the use of antiquated and often irrelevant concepts has too much impact on social, political, and economic focuses, including those that determine health care resourcing and the justification of reimbursement for medical assistance. These have raised real barriers against the individualization and personalization of management. For example, how often are bodily "impairments" the basis for defining and permitting or disallowing treatment based on the diagnostic criteria for *acute* and *chronic* medical conditions? Today, control of the "bottom line," not the benefit potential and independent achievable outcomes, is the regulator of medical and health restorative care and rehabilitation.

Comparison of Rehabilitation and Acute and Chronic Care

Unfortunately, many aspects of the restoration to a healthy state and the adaptations needed in an appropriate rehabilitative process are inconsistent with today's medical and economic controls, which are imbedded in "curable," "noncurable," "acute," or "chronic" care concepts and practices; financing limitations; outcome intentions; and so on. Direct medical services and arrangements for "health"-restorative and rehabilitative efforts require a personalized orientation and the implementation of an individualized, multiprofessional, technical and environmental adjustment program. This program may ultimately use home support persons trained and supervised by the person with severe disability instead of expensive and often unnecessary and prolonged home nursing "care."

Yet, the duration and kind of care are often limited by outcome definitions of the *curable* and *noncurable* aspects of illnesses, injuries, and defects. Exclusion of or inattention to the appropriate prevention and management of the various causes of disability and handicap, holding potential for great social and economic consequences, is discouraging, to say the least. In addition, the lack of early recognition, prevention, or remediation of preventable or treatable somatic and behavioral complications and of medical and family social attitudes often lead to pervasive, needless, and hopeless attitudes in the affected person, his or her family, and, too often, the physician. This state of affairs is augmented by the diagnosis of a noncurable pathology, such as paralysis or multiple amputations, and a hopeless prognosis for the resumption of activities of daily living. The quick results are the unmanaged disabling medical and psychosocial complications of inactivity, immobility, personal and social deactivation, and continual physical dependency. This failure to understand, encourage, and stimulate the remarkable intrinsic *adaptability* of any person having or facing severe disability is inexcusable today.

The principles for the rehabilitation of the elderly have been derived from experiences in organized programs and special centers where coordinated evaluation, treatment, and research have been dictated by the clinical problems encountered. These perspectives, very different from those in typical acute and chronic care, have emerged from the management of persons with poliomyelitis, in work with some from its onset and with others who have had it for a while. These experiences were later incorporated into organized programs for persons of all ages with spinal cord and head injury, strokes, and progressive neuromuscular and musculoskeletal disorders that had resulted from disease, injury, or defects.

These rehabilitative efforts included modifications of home conditions and community situations. These modifications were essential to assist persons with severe trauma of the nervous system, those with various acute musculoskeletal disorders, and those with degenerative neuromuscular diseases and defects. It became readily apparent that early rather than late comprehensive management leads to important benefits in outcome effectiveness and benefits in minimizing disability, dependency, and loss of autonomy.

Need to Change Attitudes toward Disability

We can no longer ignore disability or the failure to control it. Today, the survival of legions of persons from trauma and the effects of a prolonged existence are our largest causes of disability. For example, trauma in children and young adults under the age of forty-four produces more years of life lost and disability years than heart disease, cancer, and stroke. In addition, the increasing proportion of those living to eighty-five and beyond, with the concomitant frailties of advanced age, vastly increases dependency.

There will not be a vaccine or a genetic alteration in the future for the control of all the circumstances embracing trauma and aging in all its consequences. The behavior of the person, the vehicle, the driving environment, the actions of others in risk taking, and so on, will remain causative factors in auto crashes. Frail elderly persons will become totally dependent and shunted out of society into custodial warehousing as a result of appropriate and often heroic medical and surgical management *unless* they are followed up with an opportunity to resume an independent lifestyle. We can no longer fail to control, where possible, severe disability in both groups of persons.

Appropriate early management is the key to the restoration of hope and function. Contact with other persons "in the same boat" who have achieved a useful life demonstrates the real potential to achieve autonomy. The empathetic physician who sets realistic day-by-day goals and the patient's inspiration to strive ensured by his or her opportunity for autonomy have many beneficial effects. These include providing the disabled person with a sense of dignity.

The despair often engendered by disability and long-term care with dependency may be replaced by a process of restoration of healthful biological and psychological well-being coupled with rehabilitation for the resumption of functional performance in activities of daily life. Transitional opportunities to use renewed capabilities, along with the control of environmental handicaps, results in restitution of an independent lifestyle.

These interactive elements of restorative medicine and comprehensive rehabilitation are essential complements of the appropriate early treatment of pathophysiology, which, alone, may be insufficient. Even some of the most severely disabled persons succeed in attaining autonomy and independence. The addition of technical aids for mobility, communication, environmental control, home modification, and in-home attendant support help in dressing, bathing, and other care, is often a feasible substitute for expensive custodial home care. The disabled person's potential may be realized if there is community access and an opportunity to participate in community life.

A Spectrum of Health Care

In acute medicine, the causes of impairments are well known to physicians. The same is true of the pathophysiology, or disease mechanism in various organs and organ systems, that affects a person's functioning, such as loss of control of movement as the result of a stroke. In public health, there is an appropriate new emphasis on primary and secondary prevention, because trauma and various defects and other "noncurable" conditions increasingly afflict people. As indicated previously, early intervention as a form of secondary prevention and control of disability is most important in minimizing the impact of disabling impairments.

It is useful to consider the spectrum of activities that, in many instances, should replace the classic segmentation of acute and long-term care for persons facing disability. Many physicians and laypersons have recognized or are now recognizing a sequence of stages in health care in a broad and complete sense.

Health preservation today thus includes far more than absence of illness or injury. It means a system of opportunities of living in community facilities, including one's own home, that sustain physical and, frequently, emotional well-being. Such living facilities are designed to be barrier-free and to promote autonomy and independent lifestyles. They take into consideration the physical conditions and environmental opportunities needed at various ages. These are exemplified in advanced city planning, and in communities designed for elderly persons and, very recently, for the handicapped and children and youth.

Health maintenance was pioneered by the founder of the Kaiser Foundation's prepaid health-care system. Dr. Sidney Garfield developed, in parallel with typical medical-care facilities, counseling and screening for the prevention or early detection of disease, poor health habits, life stresses, and so on. His classic distinction of the "sick, the worried well, and the well" prompted health-promotional services that evolved into health maintenance in a broader sense than mere absence of illness. Also, programs for prenatal counseling, nutritional management, and so on, were provided the clients of this predecessor health maintenance organization (HMO).

Although HMOs and PPOs (preferred-provider organizations), as organized, "managed" systems of acute and chronic medical care, have proliferated over the years, they have often failed to provide restorative medicine and comprehensive rehabilitation. There is little or tardy emphasis on the preservation of biological and emotional well-being and functional performance capabilities.

Restorative medicine involves a sequence of events and styles of intervention that go into the process of acute medicine, but beyond classic diagnosis and treatment. Here, there is attention to the interaction between the person facing disability and early medical care and the influences of the social, physical, and behavioral environment of the hospital and rehabilitation center on the control of disability. We cannot stop being actively involved after proper diagnosis and acute treatment are completed.

We need first to prevent or minimize disabling medical complications and control their functional consequences. The effects of early inactivity and immobility on various bodily systems can often be prevented or minimized. Typical disabling medical problems include the development of cutaneous pressure sores; musculoskeletal problems involving loss of strength, muscular atrophy, and connective tissue contractures; and pain caused by prolonged immobility. Less obvious accompanying problems need attention, too, such as a negative nitrogen balance, subtle cardiorespiratory insufficiency besides obvious failure, and the poststress liability to infection and mental depression.

We need to recognize, especially, the loss of the will to live demonstrated in severe hopelessness and the helplessness indicated by early total dependency and loss of autonomy over the simplest functions. Depersonalization in the acute-care hospital setting of intensive care further increases loss of self-esteem.

The designation *chronically incurable,* or hopeless and beyond help, is the unkindest blow to the person's ego in a time of great fragility of will and intellect, as well as of body.

These distinctions in health care are necessary because, without them, one could not appreciate the negative significance of the "acute versus chronic" dichotomy, which harks back to Marcus Aurelius's "conditions *acuticus* and *chronicus.*" It is clearly time to broaden this pervasive dichotomy in medicine. It is out of step with today's breadth of medical research and specialized professional care emphases, as well as with society's ability to actively support prevention and to offset disability and handicap.

Restorative Medicine and Comprehensive Rehabilitation

Restorative medicine begins in the early acute and postacute phases of medical care. It extends into the phase of the preservation of residual functions and bodily structures as well as the restoration of physiological homeostasis (the stability of internal bodily functions), structural integrity, and physiological and psychological capacities. It is important to prepare the patient for the future, first by reintroducing him or her to even minimal vestiges of control, as in choice of visitors, food, telephoning, reading material, and so on. This stage should include a gradual diminution of an authoritarian and condescending manner. Group arrangements with those further along in the process are exceptionally helpful in showing the patient that he or she is not alone in devastating injury and that functional progress is truly possible. The preservation of personhood, which is crucial, must begin early and involves a long and arduous process.

In the often overlapping phases of comprehensive rehabilitation, multiple medical and allied disciplines, their technologies, and their services are combined with repetitive planning activities, with the active participation of the disabled person and, at times, the family. Teamwork in this activity is not like that in football; rather, it is a joint endeavor of experienced persons sharing perspectives, changing leadership, and setting goals. Activities are changed in accordance with the ebb and flow of the person's needs, responses, problems, and accomplishments, as the team capitalizes on the patient's improved medical restoration and physical well-being. The provision of early psychological and social support is also necessary, for emotional well-being.

Meaningful and useful functional capabilities in both ADLs (activities of daily living) and IADLs (intentional activities of daily living) have been greatly improved in recent decades by rehabilitation specialists in medicine and the allied professions. ADLs include activities such as self-care, feeding, hygiene, and mobility, whereas IADLs are activities in family and social life, such as shopping, handling financial affairs, socialization with other persons, work or avocation, and recreation. These self-chosen and independent lifestyles and activities are possible for the disabled who have an opportunity to participate in community life and to live independently instead of in a custodial "chronic"-care situation.

Physical medicine and the general medical, surgical, and orthopedic technologies are routes to the restoration of physical functioning in mobility, tolerance of increasing energy expenditure, self-care, and control of the environment. Together with multiple allied professional services and assistance, the attending physician integrates and coordinates the patient's care and often determines the indications for and timing of the participation of the classical medical specialties, such as for surgical procedures.

The cooperating allied professions include nursing, physical and occupational therapy, medical social work, psychology, rehabilitation engineering, orthotics and prosthetics, speech therapy, classroom special education for the child, and vocational counseling and training for the adult (job training, retraining, placement, etc.).

The two phases, restorative medicine and the beginning of comprehensive rehabilitation, enhance the restoration of health, including a sense of physical and emotional well-being. There is often preservation of residual functions and the development of alternatives for lost functions. A self-perceived sense of autonomy is cultivated through the careful arrangement of opportunities for the disabled person to meet progressively realistic goals that he or she has helped to define and realize. This personalized and individualized process leads to the prevention of a continuing helpless and hopeless perspective.

The later phases of comprehensive rehabilitation extend into experiences that prepare the person for independent living and increased inclusion and participation in community life, as a physical environment is changed to provide more opportunities for them.

Thus, the early anticipation and provision of restorative medicine and comprehensive rehabilitation have expanded in variety and depth. Physical and psychosocial rehabilitation have become broader and more effective in restoring functions and the capability to perform appropriately in some important aspects of daily life.

New technologies for enhanced mobility—for example, motorized triwheelers, wheelchair-accessible vans, wheelchair-accessible buses, and accommodation to the sensory losses of blind and deaf persons—will expand the opportunities for community inclusion. Accessible toilets in public facilities and sidewalk ramping, voice and Braille coding of elevator controls for the blind person, and television captioning for the deaf person have also opened up new opportunities.

Independence and Community Living

The recognition of the need to provide transitional living experiences for people who are severely impaired and handicapped but otherwise healthy followed the realization that they are capable of improved functioning and meaningful performance in life. The experiences of the 1950s and 1960s with severely disabled respirator-dependent persons revealed the need to provide a stage of group living after hospitalization as a prelude to home placement.

The question that came up later concerning many other severely handicapped persons was: How can the functional gains from institutional rehabilitation be used in community life and independent living? The better and increased use of the new mobility and environmental-control devices (such as orthotic and prosthetic devices, home revisions, and the increased availability of wheelchair-accessible transportation) noted above highlighted the social and physical barriers existing in the community. The use of physiological substitutes, such as implanted respiratory pacemakers, made possible the realization of full vocational rehabilitation for those formerly confined to nursing homes or hospitals. Simple home help in dressing and bathing and in getting in and out of vans is not only feasible for independent living but is far less costly than nursing-home care and medically oriented home care.

At first, a few new apartments were designed for the access of the disabled, as well as accommodations in local universities, and there was increased demand and justification for special public transportation in selected areas. Several special accessible and functional housing units for the severely physically handicapped were developed in some communities.

Through advocacy efforts and evidence of the value of the training of disabled persons to help others like themselves to live independently and successfully, states and the federal government have provided support for rehabilitation. Since the early 1970s, new legal authorizations have occurred in some states and the federal government, and small appropriations for independent-living support have been made available to state vocational rehabilitation agencies.

Peer counseling, personalized home-support systems, and the training of home helpers for persons facing handicaps have been developed. The appropriate supervision of home help by those being aided has become a substitute for professional nursing care. This development has been most important. Community-based, independent-living-support programs operated by and for handicapped persons as independent-living centers now number more than four hundred nationwide. These are based on pioneering models in California, Texas, Michigan, and Massachusetts.

Yet, full access to community life, including vocational and recreational opportunities, awaits the expansion of civil rights. The American Disabilities Act, signed into law by President Bush in 1991, should close the gaps. Greater access to public transportation, jobs, recreation, and housing should become the final step in the resumption of personhood and the preservation of inclusion in community life for many persons. Their only expectations in the past would have been warehousing in a confined setting. The resourcing, financing, and increased access await not only (economies of scale,) educational revision, and personnel training, but wider public realization of the hidden catastrophe of disability at all ages.

The realization of every person's potential for productivity and meaningful participation in a great and "caring" society is an overwhelmingly important goal. The constant increase in human interdependency requires the full availability of all human potential. The spirit to survive, as well as strength of willpower and resolve, remains among the great ennobling characteristics of free men and women and is a force for change.

Implications of the Failure to Provide Restorative Medicine and Comprehensive Rehabilitation

The expectation that more comprehensive rehabilitation for those facing disability is too costly is a common and incorrect viewpoint. With long-term care and the costly effects of full-blown disability and handicap, society is left, in any case, to bear the burdens of dependency. These effects include multiple hospitalizations for costly treatment of preventable complications like pressure sores, as well as the provision of prolonged custodial nursing-home care at often devastating personal and public expense. Although managed medical care, prepaid systems, and reimbursement cost controls have been popularized privately, publicly, politically, and administratively, disability benefits are often ignored in terms of rehabilitation.

Trying to save costs in early disease detection and treatment or by controlling the use of care facilities without controlling the disability and the dependency it produces will surely be counterproductive. In many instances, both the short- and long-term consequences of disabling medical complications from lack of early intervention and secondary prevention of disability have not been adequately evaluated. Exceptions include worker's compensation insurance carriers and the casualty insurance of reinsurers. They have demonstrated the cost-effectiveness of early detection and treatment: Eight to ten dollars are saved for every dollar spent.

The lesson in a multisponsored and yet incomplete health care system is often evident both to the patient and to the professionals involved in her or his care. Unless the sponsor bears the full financial burden of the failure to control disability, there is little incentive or ability to minimize a disability by providing appropriate services up front. Well-defined "health-care" sponsorship limitations (hidden rationing) are quite clear examples of curtailing the prevention and control of disability that exist in typical health insurance policies and prepaid-system reimbursements. These ostensibly emphasize cost control in order to compete with other sponsors and to minimize the cost that the employer and employee will bear in health care coverage. Thus, the view is often that the problem of disability prevention and treatment is someone else's. Actually, a sequence of cost dumps occurs. These ultimately hit (1) the taxpayer by overloading tax-supported charity hospitals; (2) the employer, in the cost of lost productivity and ever-rising medical-care expenditures; and (3) the community, the state, and the nation in the cost of long-term care unavoided and of repeated publicly sponsored hospitalizations under Medicaid, because of the lack of control of the preventable complications suffered by those impoverished by disability.

The elderly person and his or her overburdened surviving spouse and family end up as caretakers of nearly three-fourths of all those who are dependent and who are over sixty-five years old. Paradoxically, we all cry out about the rising costs of health care at the same time that we fail to stem cost-effectively the tide of increasing dependency resulting from trauma and the disabling conditions suffered by many older persons. Appropriate health-restorative care and rehabilitation would diminish the social and economic burdens of many of these consequences of a fragmented and incomplete system of care. The savings would help to control our ever-rising total health-care costs by lessening the amount of acute and critical care and decreasing disability benefit payments. A graduated redirection of expenditures to means of controlling disability and its dependency is not likely to increase the total of health-care expenditures. In the worst case, it would at least stem the rise.

The benefit and cost of realizing the full human potential and productivity achieved over a lifetime (although not considered in all of today's econometric models) should not be ignored in the future. All of this points up poignantly our need to deal with the psychosocial problem of our general unwillingness to anticipate the inevitability of disability and handicap. We need to heed the voices and experiences of various groups of the disabled who have substantiated the potential that is being lost. We are not perceiving, to the extent necessary, our capacity to deal effectively with trauma and the disabling problems of elderly persons. These problems include cost effectiveness and the yield of high self-care levels. We need far more research and development on the means of controlling disability and on making them available. Medical research in molecular biology as the panacea for the prevention of illnesses seems to be the answer proposed for most medical problems. This research is more publicly and politically appealing, as indicated by the relative expenditures of the public research-and-development dollar. However, without an equalization of the current dollar ratio of 1000 to 1 in expenditures on basic research in health and on trauma prevention and control of disability, future improvement is unlikely.

In addition, revisions in medical education are essential in this developing field of the preservation and restoration of health. Alan Gregg, a medical school dean, has said that "changing the medical school curriculum is attended by all the enthusiasm of moving a cemetery!" Surely, the dichotomies of acute and chronic, of short-term and long-term, deserve burial in the century ahead. They must be replaced by a renaissance of comprehensive and integrated individual treatment for control of disability. We need this reeducation to overcome the social and environmental as well as the physical and fiscal problems we face because of the traditional emphases in funding, educational resources, service facilities, and so on.

Implications of Advancing Age and Dependency

The associated disabling effects of aging clearly augment the consequences of our lack of resources and preparation for the onslaught of dependency that we will face in the new century.

In a lecture at the American Congress of Rehabilitation, Irving Zola, a sociology professor at Brandeis, described the increasing survival and longevity of infants and children with manifest chronic impairments, of the young adult spinal-cord and head-injured, like himself, from World Wars I and II, and of those who have experienced trauma from other causes:

> With medical advances increasing the survival of those with many chronic diseases once thought inevitable to cut short the life span, . . . the aging population will be even more at risk for what once was thought "natural" occurrences (e.g., decreases in mobility, visual acuity, hearing) and for other musculoskeletal, cardiovascular and cerebrovascular changes whose implications are only beginning to be appreciated.

> Moreover, in absolute numbers, all census data affirm that the fastest growing segment of the U.S. population is made up of those over the age of 65. In 1880 their number was less than 2 million (3%) of the total population, but by 1980 it was more than 25 million (11.3%). By the year 2030 an estimated one in four or five citizens (20 to 25%) is likely to be over 65. Put another way, throughout most of history only one in ten people lived past 65; now nearly 80% do. This traditional benchmark of 65, however, is deceptive, for the most phenomenal growth will be in the even older age groups, those over 85. This age group, while constituting 1% of the total population in 1980, is projected at 3.5% in 2030 and more than 5% in 2050. At that time they could be nearly a quarter of all elderly people. The service implications are worth noting, for, while 3% to 5% of those 65 to 74 require assistance in basic activities of daily living, more than one-third do so by age 85.[1]

When we put these comments in perspective, trauma fatalities are a greater cause of millions of years of life lost and millions of years of disability among children and adults under the age of forty-four than are heart disease, cancer, and stroke combined. *The future impact of disability is formidable if we intend to control the resulting dependency.*

Overlap between Chronic Care and Rehabilitation

The increasing burden of "chronic illness"—especially on a surviving family member, often a female spouse or younger family member, who becomes overburdened—coupled with inadequate health insurance for respite and for those providing home ADL help or home medical care, is well recognized by our aging population. The press, news magazines, and television have effectively propagated the growing social and economic crisis of aging. There is far less explicit information about available and accessible services and assistance from an organized system for health preservation, health maintenance with suitable housing, secondary prevention of disability, and comprehensive rehabilitation. The rehabilitation services covered by

Medicare have been tied primarily to particular allied professional help, such as nurses and physical therapists in the nursing homes. To a smaller degree, until very recently, a similar limitation existed in state-based Medicaid programs.

The National Institute on Aging and Human Development, together with the Institute of Medicine (IOM) of the National Academy of Science and various congressional and administrative agencies of the federal government, has issued numerous studies and reports about the growing crisis.

Pathophysiological disturbances, such as hemiplegia, have been effectively identified and managed by clinician researchers in physical medicine and rehabilitation and in geriatric medicine. An organ system approach has been emphasized for the management of cardiovascular, respiratory, metabolic, and nutritional disorders; diabetes; and osteoporosis.

The rehabilitative processes, home support, home revisions, and so on, are potent ways to diminish the need for medical care and to reduce rehospitalizations and long intervals of nursing-home placement for preventable complications.

Rehabilitative alternatives that allow continued living at home and that diminish the need for medical "care" and long-term care are likely to expand in the future because they are effective in preserving the health of elderly persons and of the family members on whom they depend. These alternatives are also more cost-effective.

Similarities and Differences of the Disabled Young and Elderly

It is helpful to examine the differences in potential and in concerns among younger persons and the elderly, especially the "frail elderly." The traumatic effects of falls, metabolic and cardiorespiratory disorders that limit physical activities, and the effects of the inactivity and immobility attendant on prolonged bed rest are disabling complications that increase in prevalence as people age. The elderly so affected are often in nursing homes or are home-bound. Many deserve to be provided earlier restorative care and rehabilitation. Some do receive the benefit of components of the rehabilitation process. We should, however, distinguish the value and differences in the appropriate use of the modalities of rehabilitation, such as physical therapy, occupational therapy, and comprehensive rehabilitation that supports independent living. These uses of different services should not be confused with the individualized and comprehensive process described above or with the potential for benefit even for those facing or having severe disability and handicaps. A piece of the process alone is not sufficient; however, there is value in any effort to restore motor function, to eliminate contractures, to improve recovery from bed sores, and to increase ambulation, for example.

The acute chronic dichotomy may undervalue the potential of benefitting from attaining and maintaining independent living and a good quality of life. This augments confusion about the choice and delivery of appropriate comprehensive services and assistance. The incredible impact on family life, socialization, and loss of organ-system coping responses to the stress of injury or disease often remains unprevented.

Table 1 contrasts some important differences between young adults and the elderly and provides a framework within which to understand the various aspects of restorative medicine and comprehensive rehabilitation previously described.

Concept and Reality of Personhood and Implications for the Physician

Given the preceding elements, the fundamental *preservation of personhood* becomes a most important aspect of the restoration of health in a broad sense of comprehensive rehabilitation in particular. It has become the touchstone of successful adaptation and life performance for the person facing disability and handicap and of the preservation of health for the elderly person. This is more than a concept. It is a practical aspect of the sense of being in control of one's life and thereby of having beneficial

Table 1. Comparison of Disability Concerns of Young Adults and the Elderly

Youth and adult perspectives	Elderly concerns
Personal and psychosocial	
Acuteness of lifestyle change to physical dependency—mourning	Anxiety about physical and social dependency on a spouse or daughter
Loss of physical attractiveness, social contacts, potential to procreate or marry, loss of breadwinner status	Suddenness of role reversal—more devastating to men
Anxiety about future life role	Fear of sudden illness and lack of ready access to help
Being forced into a nursing home, a "sick care" place with no social life appropriate to age	Potential loss of financial resources and home because of large medical care and support costs
Loss of deep friendships and normal community socialization and activity	Nursing home as a last resort and loss of all autonomy, to be cloistered with the demented and the dying
	Loss of physical mobility for shopping, socialization, recreation, etc.
Biological effects	
Extensive immobility—effects on the fit person; lessened effects on the unfit	Sedentary physiological behavior unless assisted to have heightened adaptive capacity
Significant recuperative and adaptive capability in a shorter time	Prolonged recuperative timetable and liability to disabling complications
Quicker resumption of nitrogen balance and resistance to infection	Higher incidence of secondary incapacitating illness, infections, pressure sores, etc.
Capability of building endurance and strength	Diminished physiological reserves for endurance
Greater incidence of trauma in physical activities than occurs among peers	More susceptibility to painful biomechanical stress in physical activities

biological, psychological, and social benefits. Personhood is crucial at every stage of restoration and rehabilitation.

In my opinion, this elemental drive for the preservation of personhood by each of us is responsible for the ultimate restoration of even biological well-being. It is clearly crucial because rehabilitation begins and ends with personal goals, and it therefore greatly affects the development of the potential capabilities of the person facing disability and handicap. This has been true throughout human history. The patient's perception of the possibility of achieving fulfillment despite a disability is the crucial motivation for her or his trying restorative medicine and comprehensive rehabilitation, and often for succeeding. This appears to be a fundamental example of the drive for autonomy and control of one's life, for the pursuit of happiness, and independence, for being permitted to succeed and fail, and for always being included in the community as a participant.

This drive imposes important restraints on the behavior of the physician and all others attempting to treat, assist, and support the person we identify as a "patient." His or her early drastic frality because of a major and sudden life insult so threatens the sense of self and personhood that the early contacts become pacesetters for future behaviors. This behavior can be switched from an early understanding of the necessity of compliance with the "treatment" regime to the later preservation of autonomy as a reward for personal effort and perseverance in achieving difficult biological and sociological adaptations.

The relationship of the professional to the patient must change perceptibly to one of understanding, support, and caring. The patronizing attitude of the physician—first, as director of all events in the institutional phase of treatment and, later, in dealing with extensive life adjustments—must be toned down or suppressed. This patronizing attitude may also decimate interprofessional relationships and the teamwork and leadership potential of the other professionals and technicians involved in various aspects of the total process. This process should track the dynamic changing responses and behavior of the person with the disability. The physician's recognition that the best laid plans of management are worthless if the person—or the family—is unconvinced and uncooperative is far more important than an overweening sense of being in control. Success is not always possible, but I was reassured many years ago by a great leader, Will Clayton, a former undersecretary of state, who once said that this process often succeeds because "through history the greatness of man has come from overcoming adversity."

Conclusions and Summary

The physician's role in the restorative and rehabilitative process is pivotal in protecting and sustaining the feasibility of an autonomous and independent lifestyle. He or she should recognize the need and potential for benefit of appropriate processes of rehabilitation, in guiding the patient's access to them, and in promoting the availability of the services and supports as well as providing some of the elements of the process in the appropriate contexts and at the proper time.

The practice role of the physician is definitive in the sense of integrating and supporting changes in medical management, in supporting teamwork, and in regulating the intervention of medical specialists, as well as in encouraging the leadership of various allied professionals as the status and focus of the disabled person's rehabilitation process changes.

The physician's role, like the changing status of the disabled person in rehabilitation, may vary from direct intervention in the control and management of disabling medical impairments to offering a thorough understanding of the indications for rehabilitative services and the use of the services of appropriate allied professional providers.

Physicians need to combat the understandable sense of defeat that they may feel in the face of noncurable conditions and need to associate themselves with successfully rehabilitated persons, to share their perspective and sample their successes in life and living. As a solace for failure, it is also rewarding to help others who do succeed in gratifying life adjustments.

Physicians must vigilantly face the challenge and importance of moving away from a relationship of control and an appearance of condescension in the earliest phase of dealing with their and the patient's emotional response to severe disability and loss of autonomy. Nurturing the seeds of dignity, self-respect, and potential for regaining control of one's life requires diligent attention. This can be far more helpful than unexpressed empathy. This "art" of medicine remains crucial in a doctor/patient relationship. To act otherwise is to set the stage for later animosity and lack of follow-through on the evident need for guidance in self-management by the disabled and handicapped person.

Although some medical impairments are clearly progressive and cannot be controlled, they should not limit the interim use of helpful services and supports that may ameliorate the impact of the disability on the person and the family.

There is an urgent need for medical reeducation, based on personal practice, that incorporates new concepts, knowledge, and technologies concerning the control of disability. Physicians and patients face a society unwilling to prepare for the impact of disability until it strikes home; an unprepared society will continue to lose an important national resource.

I find more and more of the elements of personalization, including talking in depth with the patient and a careful examination of the patients, to be set aside in favor of biochemical and imaging "rounds." Although these are great advances and most useful, a personal relationship remains the bridge across which the great scientific achievements must pass to be accepted and understood by the patient and, indeed, if their potential guidance to specific therapy is to be realized and appreciated.

Note

1. I. K. Zola, "Aging, Disability and the Home Care Revolution," 39th Stanley Coulter Lecture, 66th Annual Session, American College of Rehabilitative Medicine, San Antonio, Texas, November 8, 1989. Published in *Archives of Physical Medicine and Rehabilitation*, 71:2 (February 1990), p. 93.

3

"The Chaise Breaks Down, but Doesn't Wear Out"

The Goals of Geriatric Dentistry

SAUL KAMEN, D.D.S., F.A.C.D.

The title of this chapter is derived from a poem that many may remember as required reading in the fifth grade in public school. It is entitled "The Deacon's Masterpiece, or The Wonderful One Hoss Shay" and was written about 140 years ago by a prominent Boston physician, Oliver Wendell Holmes; it describes a coach that, unlike modern vehicles with their built-in obsolescence, lasted without repairs for 100 years to the day and then disintegrated. It is a long poem that I am proud to say I memorized *in toto* and recited to a public school assembly, to the enthusiastic applause of my parents and one or two others in the audience. The section most pertinent to our discussion goes as follows:

> Now in building of chaises, I tell you what,
> There is always *somewhere* a weakest spot,
> In hub, tire, felloe, in spring or thill,
> In panel, or crossbar, or floor or sill,
> In screw, bolt, thoroghbrace, lurking still,
> Find it somewhere you must and will,
> Above or below, or within or without,
> And that's the reason, beyond a doubt,
> A chaise *breaks down*, but doesn't *wear out*.

This poem is more meaningful to me now than when I recited it some sixty-five years ago because it makes two essential points—which may have been unintentional prescience on Dr. Holmes's part—about current basic concepts in gerontology and gerodontics. One is the concept of the *compression of morbidity,* which states that people today are living longer and are relatively healthy until the last three to five years of their life span, at which time they experience a cascading disease process that ultimately leads to their demise, and they then fall apart like the deacon's one-hoss shay. The second phenomenon is the astounding fact that we know enough today to enable most people to keep their natural dentition, despite some wear and tear, throughout their entire life span. This is an almost miraculous reversal of the situation that existed before World War II.

Before World War II

In the early 1940s, 10 percent of potential recruits for the U.S. Army were rejected because they could not meet the requirement of having at least six opposing natural teeth in occlusion. A recent study of the National Institute of Dental Research (NIDR) reported on the dental status of twenty-one thousand adults ranging in age from 18 to 103 years. In contrast to almost fifty years before, this study, "The National Survey of Oral Health in U.S. Employed Adults and Seniors: 1985–1986," revealed an almost complete absence of edentulism, the loss of all teeth, in persons under forty years old. Further, only 4 percent of working adults under sixty-five years old were completely without teeth, and half had lost a single tooth at most. This finding reflects the impact of dental research on the prevention of dental disease and on clinical practice in the past half century.

For many older Americans who grew up before World War II and did not benefit from prevention programs, the picture was very different. The NIDR study compared sixteen thousand working adults under sixty-five with five thousand older patients in senior citizen centers and other ambulatory elder-care agencies. In the latter group, 43 percent had lost all their teeth, a disturbing fact despite a reduction of 10 percent from previous studies conducted in the early 1970s. Although both groups had decay of the upper portion of the crown of the tooth, the older age group had three times more decay occurring at the junction of the crown and the gum than the younger group. Both groups showed a significant amount of periodontal disease and inflammation of the gingiva and supporting structures of the teeth, with increasing severity in the older age group.

(Parenthetically, another NIDR survey of children's oral health in 1986–1987 brought the good news of a dramatic decline in the caries rate in schoolchildren aged five to 17, a further sign that Americans, in general, are experiencing better dental health than did their predecessors in the first half of this century.)

Why Geriatric Dentistry?

Oral disease in older persons differs from that in younger individuals, although across generations good oral health is essential for the basic functions of chewing and speech as well as for good appearance and self-esteem.

Geriatric dentistry, lagging somewhat behind medicine in its origins, had its beginnings about a quarter of a century ago with the organization of the American Society for Geriatric Dentistry and the publication of a gerodontic journal. Paradoxically, it deals with the oldest patient population but is the youngest subdiscipline of the dental profession. Its development has been driven by the same demographic factors of aging that have influenced the direction of other professions in academic and clinical practice.

Although dentists have always treated older patients, advances in dentistry and the increase in the aging population, particularly in the past half century, led to the emergence of gerodontics, which may be defined as the science and clinical practice of providing maintenance and/or restorative and preventive oral health services to elderly patients.

Oral health care of the elderly is often complex and complicated. Besides undergoing the psychological and social deficits associated with aging, many elderly have multiple medical problems, take several medications, and have unique, age-related oral needs. These and other problems often create barriers to access to services and render a significant number of the dependent aging population at higher risk for dental problems.

As people age, their oral health has a greater impact on their lives than may be apparent. Poor oral health among the elderly often results in an unhappy concatenation of events, for example, nutritional deficiencies, metabolic disorders, and even the subtle onset of depression. In the latter stages of life, the activities of daily living often revolve around the three square meals necessary to sustain life itself. If older people retain more of their natural teeth, they become more conscious of their appearance; their self-esteem is enhanced. Recognizing that phenomenon, the University of Michigan School of Dentistry made geriatric history in 1989 by offering a program in orthodontics for the geriatric patient.

Dental Problems of Aging

Recent investigations have focused on the nature of dental disease in advancing age and have changed some of our concepts of the normal and pathological effects of aging on dentition.

Significant differences have been described in the oral mucous membranes of individuals younger than sixteen and those over sixty, including an increase in hardening of the cell membrane surrounding the teeth and gums and a thinning of the tissue. Although some question these differences, the empirical evidence can be readily confirmed, particularly in the toothless patient, by experienced prosthodontists and oral pathologists. It is probably correct to ascribe these changes to disease or pharmacological intervention, but there is no doubt that these changes are also part of the progressive catabolic processes of ischemia and nitrogen imbalance, although there are always exceptions.

Oral motor behavior includes the posture of the lips and the orofacial musculature, mastication, swallowing, speech, and sensorimotor skills. All, which have an impact on quality of life, decline with aging.

Other studies on relatively healthy dentate individuals conclude that, in these subjects, masticatory effort—that is, the ability to chew a wad of food—does not change significantly with age, but that masticatory efficiency, the time required to chew food in preparation for swallowing, increases in older age groups. These studies also showed a distinct correlation between the number of teeth lost or missing and the acceptability of certain foods. Another longitudinal study of an essentially healthy elderly population residing in Baltimore confirmed these findings of diminished chewing efficiency and also found diminished capacity of function-lip posture, tongue stability, and swallowing.

Catabolic effects, or the destructive metabolic effects of aging on the soft tissues of the mouth, may include dehydration, mineral imbalances, peripheral ischemia, and changes in the bacterial flora. These conditions then result in a higher incidence of lesions of the oral mucous membranes. Another common marker of aging is a less efficient immune system. As a consequence, many elderly are prone to candidial, or fungal, infections of the mouth. Other conditions that occur with greater frequency among the elderly include inflammatory viral herpetic and blistering lesions of the tissues lining the mouth.

Dry Mouth Problems

Two disorders that are particularly common among and predominantly affect the elderly deserve special attention. They are xerostomia, or dry mouth, and "burning-mouth syndrome."

The diagnosis of xerostomia is essentially a subjective clinical evaluation. Though many elderly patients learn to endure the symptoms without complaint, dry mouth can affect speech, taste, nutritional behavior, and retention of dental prostheses. As the amount of saliva decreases, plaque builds up more rapidly and tooth enamel is less resistant to decay; the result is more dental caries, periodontal disease, and candidial conditions.

Xerostomia may have many underlying causes, ranging from the large quantity of drugs prescribed for elderly patients to systemic conditions such as diabetes and some arthritic conditions. Whatever the cause, the preventive management of dry mouth requires cooperation among all caregivers, including physicians, dentists, and nursing staff. If psychotropic drugs are the cause, family and social support will be especially necessary.

Basic strategies for the management of xerostomia include:

- Enhanced oral hygiene measures, including topical fluorides, to reduce the colonization of bacterial organisms and the proliferation of oral pathogens.
- Utilization of water, 10 percent glycerin solution, or over-the-counter artificial saliva substitutes.
- Utilization of sialogogues, agents that promote the flow of saliva, which are currently undergoing extensive research at the National Institute of Dental Research. These medications must be appropriately administered and supervised by the patient's dentist.
- Daily application of topical fluoride gels for patients scheduled for radiation therapy to the head and neck before, during, and after radiotherapy. Such patients should be screened, and nonrestorable teeth should be extracted before irradiation.

"Burning Mouth"

A baffling disorder that occurs more prominently after the fifth decade of life is burning-mouth syndrome. Although some consider it to be a stress-related condition with a strong psychogenic component, it is a complex problem reflecting many catabolic changes in aging. Intense pain is accompanied by a dry mouth and hypersensitivity of the oral mucosa, which may appear inflamed or pale and anemic. A detailed drug profile should be elicited, as the elderly are particularly prone to adverse reactions. In most cases, palliative treatment should be vigorously undertaken. Treatment would include:

- Use of artificial saliva as needed.
- Swishing for one minute with a mouthwash consisting of equal parts of elixir of Benadryl and Kaopectate, then expectorating. This should be prescribed and supervised by the patient's dentist.
- Use of 2 percent viscous Xylocaine (lidocaine) for recalcitrant cases, prescribed and supervised by the patient's dentist.
- Referral for psychological or psychiatric consultation.

Medical and Dental Interdependence

As is apparent from the foregoing discussion, oral health and general physical health are closely intertwined. The past fifty years have taught us that the impact of poor oral health on the clinical management of geriatric patients can seriously compromise progress and alter prognosis. For example, an impaired ability to chew may thwart efforts to provide proper nutrition for the victim of a stroke. Similarly, lack of compliance with the guidelines of the American Heart Association has been identified as the chief causal factor in subacute endocarditis (inflammation of the heart lining) when the cardiac patient has not used the recommended antibiotic prophylaxis before the intervention.

As the elderly are increasingly integrated into dental practice, the physician will be called on more frequently for advice on such diverse aspects of care as the drug profile of the patient and the possible contraindication of certain dental procedures. The physician will need to be consulted about prescribing sedatives for patients with depression or dementia and about how best to deal with oral manifestations caused by medical treatment.

Medical-Dental Interfaces

The older patient with medical problems may be at higher risk for dental care than the relatively healthy person. For this reason, when an elderly individual is being treated by a physician, it is a wise policy to ask if there are any precautions that should be observed before the patient undergoes dental care. The dentist, too, should be informed by the patient of his or her medical status in great detail. It is also necessary to give the dentist a list of all medications, prescription or over-the-counter, as these may be a clue to certain conditions that may interact with dental management. I cite here just a few of the medical problems that influence dental treatment and briefly describe the medical-dental interface.

Cardiovascular Disease

The patient with cardiovascular disorders, such as myocardial infarction, coronary artery disease, or mitral valve prolapse, is at risk for an infection known as subacute bacterial endocarditis (SBE) following most invasive dental procedures. The American Heart Association has a very specific protocol of antibiotic prophylaxis that the patient and the dentist should use before dental treatment. Failure to comply with these recommendations is one of the major causes of the admission of elderly patients to hospitals for SBE following dental procedures. It may also be helpful to relieve the cardiac patient of the stress and anxiety of dental treatment by prescribing a mild sedative before the appointment.

On the other hand, it is important that the dentist should consult with the patient's physician if there is any question of an interaction between the drugs that have been prescribed by the physician and the medications the dentist may wish to use, for example, local anesthetic agents. Some of the long-term drugs commonly administered to the patient with cardiac problems (e.g., digitalis) may cause nausea or even vomiting while the patient is undergoing dental treatment, but this is usually a transient episode and can be controlled by the sedative agents previously mentioned. Another precaution of which the patient should be aware is that many dentists now treat patients in a recumbent or prone position, and in the case of hypertension and concomitant drug regimens, there is a tendency for syncope (faintness) if the chair is pulled upright too quickly or if the patient is discharged before adjusting to the change. The safest rule in the dental management of cardiac patients is that the dentist should routinely consult with the physician regarding antibiotic prophylaxis and the other precautions described above.

Cerebrovascular Disorders

For the patient who has had a stroke or a related cerebrovascular disorder, there are significant considerations in undergoing dental care. First, it should be remembered that adequate nutritional support during the recovery period will often depend on good oral function. In many cases, unfortunately, the mouth is severely affected by the stroke, and masticatory ability is impaired. Therefore, the restoration of oral function is an integral component of the rehabilitation process and is often quite challenging because of neuromuscular deficiencies. In addition to the mechanical considerations in oral rehabilitation, the interaction of the anticoagulant therapy usually prescribed and dental treatment may also be hazardous to the patient. If such a patient is scheduled for oral surgery, for example, or any other dental procedure that may result in hemorrhaging, the patient's blood must be monitored before this treatment. Again, consultation between the dentist and the physician is highly recommended, indeed almost mandatory, in such cases. It is also increasingly apparent that the dentist must communicate with pharmacists, speech pathologists, and physical medicine therapists regarding his or her role in the overall strategy of rehabilitation.

Cancer

Another area where oral health geriatricians must interface with other health-care givers is in the treatment of the patient with oral cancer. It has been estimated that there are thirty thousand new cases of oral cancer each year, and nine thousand deaths, predominantly in patients over sixty years old.[1] The deleterious effect of cancer therapies on the hard and soft tissues of the mouth reflects the common adverse side effects of modalities of treatment. The subsequent impact on the quality of life has been observed in many of our nursing-home patients. A major complication is the effect of radiation therapy on the salivary glands, the muscles of mastication and deglutition, the bones of the mouth, and, ultimately, the teeth, if they are not protected against the catabolic environmental changes. Thus, it is essential that, early in the management of the cancer patient, the oncologist and radiation therapists consult with the dentist, who can prevent or ameliorate some of these adverse complications. A National Institutes of Health Consensus Development Conference, held in Bethesda, Maryland, in April 1989, recommended a specific protocol for pretherapy strategies by dentists to attenuate and alleviate the incidence and morbidity of oral complications—and sometimes mortality.

A major oral manifestation caused by chemotherapy, which is often used after cancer surgery, is the fungal infection *Candida albicans,* which may be transient or, in the severely immunocompromised patient, more persistent. In either case, we may observe inflammation of the mucosa, secondary bacterial infections, and hemorrhaging. Dental management, usually in consultation with the physician, includes the use of antifungal mouthwashes, most recently chlorhexidine gluconate and/or 10 percent clotrimazole.

Dementia

In the demented patient, the teeth may decay more rapidly than the mind, but the rung of dental care is often neglected in the ladder of services required and sought by the affected individuals and their caregivers. In fact, as the dementia progresses, the patient may forget that she or he has a mouth, much less that she or he finds it difficult to perform elementary oral hygiene. Other factors that result in rampant decay and gingival disease include dry mouth, which is an inevitable side effect of the psychotropic drugs commonly prescribed. The same medications, particularly the phenothiazines, may cause tardive dyskinesia (i.e., spastic movements of the mouth, tongue, and lips), which may result in ulcerations of the soft tissues as well as destruction of the tooth enamel. For these reasons, the dentist is compelled to consult with the psychiatrist when the symptoms are first identified. With the increasing incidence of dementia in our aging population, the role of the dental practitioner has become more clearly delineated. Geriatric dentists must be trained to recognize the onset of dementia, must be able to correlate their treatment with the stage of the disease, and must consult with other professionals regarding the management of the uncooperative and sometimes belligerent patient.

These are only some of the challenging problems in treating the multiply medically compromised older patient. It is this dilemma that often makes geriatric dentistry more touching than technological, more caring than curing, and that generates more compassion than composites.

Utilization and Cost of Dental Care

Although the oral health needs of the elderly are challenging and extensive, the NIDR study previously cited showed that the elderly are enjoying better dental health than in the past and have higher expectations for the preservation of their dentition. These facts are reflected in the increasing demand for dental care. Between 1978 and 1983, the number of dental visits of persons sixty-five and older increased by more than 40 percent. During this same five-year period, the average number of visits by older dental patients increased within the last year by 25 percent, that is, from 1.2 to 1.5 visits a year. The utilization patterns differed in those with and without teeth; more than half, or 55 percent, of those with their own teeth had visited a dentist during the past year, compared to 13 percent of older patients without teeth.

Although this pattern of increased utilization is partially the result of intensified educational efforts by national dental organizations, such as the Senior Smile Week recently initiated by the American Dental Association, the major factor in the utilization of oral health services is the affordability of care. The economic status of many of the elderly, particularly those in the sixty-five to seventy-five age group, has greatly improved. Whereas 25 percent of Americans live at or near the poverty line, this young-old group has twice the mean net worth, $125,000, of all U.S. families ($60,000). Yet the socioeconomic problems of this age group are great. One-third of the near-poor elderly are reduced to poverty by their out-of-pocket payments for medical and dental care, including long-term care.

According to a report on future health care in America by a Subcommittee on Education and Health of the U.S. Joint Economic Committee:

> In America health care is a privilege, not a right. It is costly. It is inefficient. Access is not universal. . . . As we move toward the 21st century and our population keeps aging, bold and immediate steps must be taken if inter-class and inter-generational conflict are to be averted.[2]

A 1985 study determined that seven out of ten older persons living alone could be impoverished by even a thirteen-week nursing-home stay, and that married persons "spend down" to the poverty level in twenty-six weeks of long-term care.

Dental Insurance, Medicare, and Medicaid

Although dental insurance programs have proliferated considerably throughout the United States, their benefits are primarily related to employment and cease when the covered person leaves her or his job or retires from the work force. Medicare has few dental benefits, and a 1981 amendment to the regulations of the Health Care Finance Administration (A 2020.3) allowing reimbursement for medically related oral conditions, though not direct care to the teeth, is largely ignored and underused. The American Society for Geriatric Dentistry has attempted unsuccessfully, through legislative channels, to expand dental benefits under this amendment, which includes authorizing reimbursement for new tooth-implant technology in medically related conditions.

It has been suggested that Medicare Part A and Part B should be enlarged to provide coverage for acute dental services, such as pain, infection, swelling, and other pathology of the oral tissues, based on the same rationale as that for the treatment of other health-threatening conditions. Certainly, no person, young or old, should be denied such service because of an inability to pay.

Medicaid, Title XIX of the Social Security Act of 1965, is the major source of support for dental services for low-income groups of elderly and disabled persons. Under federal rules, each state determines the eligibility of patients, the types and range of services, the fees (on either a per service or a per visit basis), and the administrative and operating procedures. Although certain services, such as inpatient and outpatient hospital care and skilled nursing care are mandated, the states may use their discretion in providing optional services such as podiatric, optometric, dental, and physical therapy, as well as items such as prescription drugs, dentures, prosthetic devices, and glasses.

For instance, Alabama, Delaware, Idaho, Texas, and Wyoming limit dental care only to children with conditions noted during early periodic screening, diagnosis, and treatment programs. Of the remaining 45 states, 30 require authorization before treatment, 42 place other limits on dental services, and dentures are provided by 38 states. Many of these programs suffer from inadequate coverage, low fee schedules, and inordinate paperwork, all of which are disincentives for the participation of dental professionals.

It may not be realistic in the present economic and political climate to press for an expansion of Medicaid benefits to meet the increasing oral needs of indigent noninstitutionalized elderly persons. William Reynolds, Director and Chief Dental Officer of the Bureau of Standards Development in the New York State Department of Health, said, however, that "a possible strategy to improve dental services is to work at the federal level to strengthen the standards in the Medicare and Medicaid Conditions of Participation as they apply to dental services in nursing homes and to strengthen the Medicare and Medicaid programs themselves."[3] To accomplish this objective, dentistry needs the support not only of allied health professionals, but of elderly dental consumers themselves, and of lay agencies concerned with the advancement of geriatric health care.

Geriatric Education

Since the early 1980s, major initiatives by government agencies have begun to meet the need to develop leadership in gerontology and geriatric education. In dentistry, the Veteran's Administration established in the early 1980s a Geriatric Dental Fellowship Program in five VA centers. This program is ongoing and has produced a cadre of well-trained professionals, many of whom are serving in academic and institutional arenas. In many state-supported medical and dental schools, as well as schools of allied health sciences, geriatrics has been mandated as a component of the predoctoral curriculum.

More recently, Congress passed the Public Health Service Act of 1987 (P.L. 100-177), which gives grants to schools of medicine and osteopathy for traineeships and fellowships to train physicians and dentists to teach geriatric medicine or geriatric dentistry. There are two tracks in this fellowship training program, now being pursued in sixteen medical centers in the United States. One is a one-year retraining program in geriatrics for physicians and dentists who are currently faculty members; the other is a one- or two-year internal medicine or family medical fellowship program. The latter is designed to provide training in clinical geriatrics and geriatric research for physicians who have completed graduate medical education and dentists who have completed postdoctoral dental education programs.

Most exciting for the dental profession is the mandate that these programs be conducted by both medical and dental faculty, and that the ultimate goal be to promote interdisciplinary leadership of professionals with exceptional competence in teaching the cognitive, attitudinal, and psychomotor skills essential to the rehabilitation and management of medically compromised older patients. The guidelines for the conduct of this program should ensure the development of future geriatricians with a keen understanding of the societal factors, socioeconomic issues, behavioral aspects of diseases of the elderly, and ethical considerations that often influence the strategies and tactics of diagnosis, management, and treatment.

Developing leadership in geriatrics in academia demands that experienced health-care professionals extend their creative talents to the task of incorporating oral health services into an interdisciplinary-care curriculum enriched with diverse clinical experience. Given these developments in academic education, it is the responsibility of the diverse organizations concerned with health care to foster and encourage legislative support on the federal and state levels for the continuation and expansion of these initiatives.

Dental Care in Nursing Homes

With the dramatic growth in the older population in the United States and the exponential increase in the oldest-old, long-term care will continue to be the most common health-care need of the aging. Gregory Pawlson, Past President of the American Geriatric Society, estimated that "we face a two-to-three fold rise in the use of hospital and physician services, and a nearly four-fold rise in the use of long term care services by the year 2040."

In terms of numbers, Robert H. Binstock, Professor of Aging, Health and Society at the Case Western Reserve School of Medicine, calculated that the current nursing-home population of 1.5 million will increase to 2.1 million by the year 2000 and will reach 4.4 million by 2040. This estimate does not include millions of noninstitutionalized people who may be severely disabled and home-bound.[4]

The history of oral health care for elderly persons in nursing-home and related domiciliary facilities is not a happy one. In the nursing-home scandal of 1975, a House Special Committee on Aging cited oral neglect among the litany of abuses of residents. Since then, the Health Care Finance Administration has tried to make adequate dental care a condition for nursing-home participation in Medicare- and Medicaid-reimbursed programs, but without much success.

Some major factors contributing to this problem have been expense, the psychosocial characteristics of the patient population, and the inadequacies of regulatory oversight. Medicaid, which is the chief source of reimbursement for dental services in the nursing-home industry, accounts for only 2 percent of the total national expenditures for dentistry, a meager allocation for institutional health care. In addition to the financial barriers to dental care for institutionalized patients, their debilitated medical status and mental incompetence often mitigate against comprehensive oral rehabilitation.

Even so, with a positive attitude of therapeutic optimism, such patients can benefit from good-quality oral health care. An enforcement of statutes already on the books is needed to raise the standards of dental care in thousands of U.S. nursing homes.

Two Dental-Health Task Forces

In 1988 and 1989, the New York State Department of Health established two task forces concerned with dental health. The first was charged with revising the operating standards for the provision of dental services in residential health-care facilities. The second included incorporating oral health care in the Implementation Manual of the New York State Quality Assurance Program. Both may serve as models for other states to follow.

In response to the Nursing Home Reform Law passed by Congress in 1987, the New York State health department issued a directive to all skilled-nursing facilities (SNFs) and health related facilities (HRFs) that all operators must provide directly, or make arrangements for, routine and emergency dental services to meet the needs of each resident. The task force assembled by the state Medicaid agency advised the department on a method of reimbursement for those services in which each facility would receive thirty to fifty cents per day per bed. In return, dental providers would be expected to deliver optimal levels of service.

These services include oral screening of all patients within four days of admission to determine conditions of an emergency nature, a more complete oral examination within thirty days of admission, in-service education programs, and timely and appropriate treatment based on the individual needs of each resident.

These regulations make the operators directly responsible for the execution of dental services and require them to submit a budget for salaries, equipment, and supplies for each facility. The plan has attracted many dental professionals and has been implemented with varying degrees of success.

The second task force dealt with the implementation of the Long Term Survey process mandated by the federal Omnibus Budget Reconciliation Act of 1987, which incorporated certain nursing-home reform amendments. Provisions related to oral health include:

- Direct observation of a random sampling of patients to determine if they have specific oral complaints and are satisfied with their dental treatment.
- An inspection of on-site dental clinics and the supplies available to the residents for daily oral hygiene.
- Confirmation that dentures have been labeled and identified (mandatory in some states).
- Systematic in-service education programs in oral health care for the nursing staff.
- A review of documents to determine that there has been interdisciplinary consultation and a consideration of each resident's physical and mental limitations of function in the design and timely performance of an appropriate treatment plan.
- Evidence of informed consent and the patients' willingness to accept treatment.

The implementation of the quality assurance process for oral health care will not be achieved unless federal and state auditors are adequately trained to evaluate these prerequisites.

Nevertheless, there are enough regulatory statutes on the books so that, if they are enforced, they will rapidly elevate the oral health status of institutionalized older patients. Realistically, we cannot expect a revolutionary change in levels of oral health care unless dentistry enlists the support of other professions and concerned lay agencies.

Recommendations

What will help the oral "chaise" of the elderly from breaking down? Here are four specific recommendations:

- Education of all of the health and health-related professions on the role of oral health in our aging population.
- Support for a continuation of the federal programs that incorporate geriatric oral health in the curricula of all undergraduate and postgraduate schools of the health professions.
- Exploration and support of measures that will expand the benefits for dental care through Medicare, Medicaid, and other third-party insurance programs.
- Support of the appropriate oral health services in the implementation of quality assurance in nursing homes and home-bound programs.

Notes

1. *Consensus Statement: Oral Complications of Cancer Therapies*. National Cancer Institute Monograph.
2. D. H. Scheur, Staff Report, Subcommittee on Health and Education of the U.S. Joint Economic Committee, October 2, 1989.
3. W. E. Reynolds, Staff Report, Subcommittee on Health and Education of the U.S. Joint Economic Committee, October 2, 1989.
4. R. H. Binstock, "Health Care for Older Populations: Society's Responsibilities," *Health Matrix* (National Publishing Company), 6:3 (1988).

Suggested Reading

S. Kamen, "Current Concepts in Geriatric Dentistry," *Current Treatment in Dental Practice,* ed. N. Levine. Philadelphia: W. B. Saunders, 1986.

"NIDR: 40 Years of Progress," *Journal of the American Dental Association,* 116 (June 1988).

4

Feet and the Aging Process

A. Podiatric Medicine and Aging

ARTHUR E. HELFAND, D.P.M.

Introduction

Foot problems in the older adult are constant. The foot undergoes a great deal of trauma, use, misuse, and neglect during life's activities. As the stresses associated with walking, activity, and mobility are coupled with the changes associated with the aging process (e.g., systemic diseases, focal or localized impairment, and environmental factors), limited mobility, discomfort, and pain may result. Some foot problems increase the risk of complications from systemic diseases and the potential for foot, or lower extremity, amputation. These conditions may affect the individual's ability to walk, to take care of herself or himself, and to remain an active, productive, independent member of society. The loss of ambulation often deprives the elderly individual of self-respect and creates social segregation, which may lead to declining health and may cause personality and emotional changes.

Comprehensive primary podiatric care, with an emphasis on prevention, is essential in keeping the elderly walking. Such care, especially during the rehabilitation period following any debilitating or deconditioning disease, is a major catalyst for motivation and health.

Factors Contributing to Foot Problems

Many factors contribute to the development of foot problems in the older patient. One of the most basic is the degree of ambulatory function—walking, running, or standing—throughout the patient's life. The stress, force of impact, and repetitive trauma associated with ambulation take a toll. Past foot conditions and/or diseases and the type of foot care services received, or the lack of them, also affect future problems. Improper footwear, incompatible in fit and/or function, is a major contributory factor, as is walking on harsh surfaces, such as concrete or stone, that have no give or resiliency.

As the individual ages, the number of factors that can cause foot problems increases. Atrophy from underuse, multiple chronic diseases, musculoskeletal diseases, and certain diseases such as diabetes mellitus complicate medical management and place the individual at risk for foot complications. These may include infection, decrease or lack of circulation, and insensitivity leading to a diminished response to pain, cold, heat, or even position. Current medications and certain therapeutic programs involving excessive exercise without adequate protection may also induce foot problems.

Many changes associated with aging (e.g., personal losses, changes in societal role, cognitive dysfunction, lessened physical function, and changes in living style) often put limitations on mobility. The emotional stress involved may also have a negative effect on foot health.

Other major factors contributing to the foot problems of the elderly are hospitalization and institutionalization. Depending on how long the patient is immobilized, hospitalization may decondition the feet and turn a minor foot problem into a major one that limits activity. And because Medicare and Medicaid offer only limited coverage of primary and preventive foot care, so that eventually some patients must needlessly enter hospitals, these federal programs, too, can be said to be contributory factors.

Podiatric Assessment

The assessment, evaluation, and examination of older patients for foot health involve more than a clinical knowledge of the foot. The examiner must recognize the patient's concerns and needs with a special emphasis on comfort. To enhance patient care, an interdisciplinary team, often including the primary physician, medical specialists, physical therapists, podiatrists, and so on, should be used, and the caregivers should agree on goals (e.g., the relief of pain and the restoration of function and functional stability). The clinician must anticipate projected changes in ambulation and foot care needs and must provide an assurance of individual dignity.

The initial element of the assessment should include demographic data and the patient's living conditions. Both the personal activities of daily living (e.g., ambulation, dressing, grooming, and bathing) and instrumental activities (e.g., shopping, housekeeping, and transportation) should be taken into consideration when one is assessing foot complaints and/or conditions.

The chief complaint and patients' perceptions of their own problems should be noted in the patients' own terms, as well as how these changes affect their daily lives and activities. Footwear should be assessed for its fit, function, use, and compatibility with foot type. The duration, location, and severity of current conditions should be noted, and prior treatment, results, and relation to other general medical conditions should be ascertained.

The patient's past foot-care history and the use of commercial foot-care products should be identified. The patient's past occupational history should be explored, including foot-related activities on the job, military service, geographic location, and percentage of weight bearing, which take into account total body weight, force on the foot in walking and standing, and the total amount of time spent in weight-bearing activities. Flooring and footwear on the job should be noted.

An anatomical systems review should be part of the history, and the vascular, neurological, musculoskeletal, and integumentary functions should be noted for each system. Current medications and responses to them should be identified, along with existing and past therapeutic programs. The past history should include infections, operations, fractures, injuries, drug sensitivities, and allergies. Those problems and diseases that have foot, or pedal, complications and/or that affect foot care and ambulation should be identified as risk factors. Such conditions are many, ranging from diabetes mellitus, arteriosclerosis, and malnutrition, to cancer, edema, leprosy, and hypertension.

Recognizing Common Foot Problems in the Elderly

Skin Conditions

The skin is one of the first structures to demonstrate age- and disease-related change. There is a loss of hair due to less efficient circulation. There is a gradual appearance of brownish pigmentation, anhidrosis (lack of sweating), and xerosis (excessively dry skin). Early fissure lines occur with prolonged periods of repeated microtrauma (wear and tear on the feet, as from pounding on a concrete sidewalk), diminished nutrition, and excessive dryness. Itching often accompanies these changes, giving rise to abrasions and other skin irritations. The initial treatment of these conditions should be hydration and lubrication.

Other skin conditions include contact dermatitis, fungal infections such as athlete's foot, and bacterial skin infections. Depending on the cause, management includes the use of topical steroids, antifungals, and antibiotics.

Given the coexistence of foot deformity and related systemic diseases, such as arteriosclerosis and diabetes mellitus in many cases, initial abrasions may result in the development of ulceration (loss of tissue), deeper infection, necrosis (death of local tissue), and the loss of a part or all of the foot. Early evaluation and intervention are keys to the reduction of complications in these foot problems in the elderly.

The Toenails

Multiple changes may take place in the toenails with aging. The contour and shape of the toenail may change, and if care is neglected, ram's horn nail, a thickening of the toenail causing deformity and enlargement, may occur. These changes are the residual of a decrease in the vascular supply to the nail bed, poor nutrition, and repeated microtrauma. When the foot is shod, there is significant continuing abrasion between the underside of the toe box and the upper surface of the toenails, resulting in continuing microtrauma. An associated fungus of the toenails increases the prevalence of the ram's horn deformity, with further thickening.

The diabetic patient often experiences a series of nail changes specifically associated with the disease: thickening of the cuticle, striations and/or transverse lines on the nail plate, an increase in callous formation, blood under the toenail, and nail deformity. Sometimes thinning of the cuticle occurs, as does involution, or a C-shaped curvature of the nail. As the normal curvature of the nail is modified, a callous may form under the nail, causing some loosening of the nail plate from the edge. Calloused nail grooves elicit pain. In conjunction with involution, pain and limitation of ambulation may occur. Continuing pressure, as from an improperly fitted shoe, can initiate ulceration of the toenail.

Management of these conditions includes periodic débridement, or surgical removal of the devitalized parts, of the nail plate; partial removal is required initially. The use of emollients to lubricate and soften callous tissue is appropriate. When the deformity continues to cause excessive pain, removal and excision of the entire nail may be indicated.

An appropriate review of the vascular and metabolic status of the patient precedes any surgical consideration. Shoes with a high toe box and protective materials such as lamb's wool and polyfoam caps help to reduce pressure on the nail plate and may minimize the need for surgical management by reducing pain and pressure. The pain and discomfort that result from these conditions and their inappropriate management limit ambulation and produce significant complications for the elderly patient.

Fungus of the toenails is another common condition in the elderly. It is related both to the invading organism and to the environmental factors associated with this chronic infection. Some of these factors are repeated microtrauma, shoe friction, and the dark, moist, warm environment within the shoe itself. If not properly treated, the superficial infection remains, and the organisms invade the nail plate top and bottom, destroying the nail plate itself. Loosening of the nail plate is common with fungus under the toenail. An increase in size (hypertrophy) often follows, along with a brownish-yellow color and a musty odor. An inflammation of the toenail can develop from continuing irritation and infection of varying degrees, sometimes including the cuticle and the surrounding tissue. Pain and discomfort usually result from hypertrophy and pressure. Surgical nail removal and disease-related nail loss are also common in the elderly and are complicating factors if early management is not provided.

Initial management in the older patient with fungal toenails should consist of periodic debridement, mild lubricants to help soften the nail beds and folds, and topical antifungal solutions that provide some stability for treatment. One must continually manage this chronic infection in order to prevent complications and provide comfort and ambulatory ability.

Structural and Organic Changes

Hyperkeratotic lesions, or hardened thick skin such as calluses and corns, are of concern to the older patient. These lesions represent both primary pathology (diseases in themselves) and symptoms of other related foot deformities. Treatment in the older patient often consists of management of the residual deformities and the related systemic diseases, such as diabetes mellitus, arterial insufficiency, and degenerative joint disease.

Hyperkeratosis is a protective mechanism that results from physical stress and acts as a space replacement when soft tissue atrophies. Hammer toes, loss of muscle mass, bunions, atrophy, decreased function, and shoe-to-foot incompatibilities tend to decrease ambulation and result in pain and discomfort. These conditions are not normal and require treatment and continuing care if the patient is to remain pain-free, comfortable, and ambulatory.

The changes in structure due to physiological change or disease that occurs in the musculoskeletal system are the primary causes of the development of areas of hardened and thickened skin, which cause the foot to increase in size, sometimes grossly, and are related to atrophy, the thinning of bone and muscle, and excessive dryness.

Functional Imbalance

Some of the conditions that precipitate pain and discomfort in the elderly are related to functional imbalance and dysfunction. That is, parts of the foot lose their ability to perform as they should because of a change in position, and the result is that the patient loses some ability to function. Hammer toes, bunions, heel spurs, and the local joint changes of arthritis and inflammation of the soft tissues, tendons, and joints are examples of some of these conditions. Each produces some degree of limitation of motion, as well as discomfort and pain. These problems are often related to inadequate, or incompatible, footwear.

Proper shoe selection, fit, and modification may be indicated and may be augmented by the use of orthotics, that is, special molds placed in the shoe to permit the foot to function more normally. These measures, along with special lasts and the fabrication of molds from some of the newer materials available, can reduce shock, minimize stress, reduce friction, and redistribute weight.

Effects of Systemic Diseases

Many systemic diseases produce serious foot complications. Osteoarthritis, or degenerative joint disease, may be a major factor in limiting walking. The primary clinical manifestations of these diseases in the elderly include inflammation of the soft tissue on the bottom of the foot, bony changes due to arthritis, spur formation, inflammation of the bone covering, and tendonitis. Fixed deformities and inflammatory reactions to repeated microtrauma produce swelling, stiffness, and pain. Management includes medication for pain, foot orthotics for increased stability, and physical therapy and rehabilitation to provide relief from the pain, restoration of function, and maintenance of mobility in the future.

The primary form of traumatic arthritis in the elderly is hallux limitus, a limitation of the range of motion at the large toe joint. As deformity and spur formation increase, the condition becomes hallux rigidus, a fixed deformity of the same joint that precludes movement. Pain results from the constant irritation. Orthotics and shoe modifications that bridge the joint and eliminate motion usually control pain and enhance ambulation. The addition of physical therapies, such as ultrasound, whirlpool, muscle stimulation, and infrared light, to assist in the management of the acute symptoms, increases foot function.

Other forms of arthritis—that is, neurotrophic (which entails changes caused by a neurological disease), infectious, gouty, and rheumatoid—lead to degenerative changes frequently present in older individuals. If there is pain, bone disintegration and osteoporosis should be considered. Neurotrophic changes are most often associated with long-standing diabetes mellitus. Acute gout gives rise to severe pain and swelling. The chronic changes of long-standing gout include urate deposits (salts from uric acid) and ulceration, as well as pronounced deformity and degeneration. The continuing use of diuretics for hypertension and cardiac disease may produce a goutlike syndrome in the elderly, with marked discomfort, pain, and limitation of ambulation. The end result of rheumatoid arthritis in the elderly includes residual deformity, atrophy, contractures, rigidity, and gait changes that add to ambulatory disability and increase the potential for falls, with all of their attendant complications.

Diabetes Mellitus

A significant number of the elderly suffer from diabetes mellitus. Many times a foot complaint or problem is the initial symptom of diabetes for which the patient seeks medical care, so that the foot condition becomes the portal of entry into the health care system. Early supportive measures can help limit future disability and reduce the possibility of severe ambulatory dysfunction in persons with degenerative changes. The manifestations of diabetes in the feet involve multiple systems and are associated with a variety of symptoms and signs, ranging from sensory impairment, motor weakness, and nerve damage, to infection, necrosis, and gangrene.

The potential for amputation of the foot increases when other conditions accompany the diabetes. These include obesity, hypertension, smoking, too much fat or sugar in the blood, and peripheral vascular disease. Neuropathy, or a change in the nervous system causing abnormal sensations, may also increase the likelihood of amputation. Other conditions that increase the potential include minor trauma brought on by faulty proprioception, or not knowing where the foot is; infection; inadequate health education; lack of preventive measures; and poor foot care. Additional risk factors include a loss of protective sensation, existing foot deformity, and a prior history of pedal ulceration.

Many factors cause diabetic ulceration to develop in the older patient, one of the most important being poor knowledge of foot care. Other factors include a period of continuous pressure and local arterial ischemia, or lack of blood from the arterial system, related to deformity and improper gait, or walk; counterpressure from a thickening of the skin; continued and repeated microtrauma; and friction, with thrusting and shearing in improperly fitted shoes. Hemorrhage under the callous or thickened skin is usually the earliest sign of impending ulceration or its potential. Coexistent changes in foot structure additionally contribute to the development of foot ulcers. When one considers the cost of a lower extremity amputation (which may result from a diabetic ulceration) for the patient, the family, and society, foot health education becomes cost-effective as an initial step in the prevention of foot loss.

Arterial Insufficiencies and the Neurological System

Peripheral arterial insufficiency, or decreased arterial blood supply, is present to some degree in most older persons. Overt indications include muscle fatigue, cramps, limping, coldness, numbness, burning, and hair loss.

Foot ulcers resulting from arterial insufficiency are usually painful and extremely slow in healing. Dry gangrene—the localized death of a foot part, usually due to lack of circulation—is characteristic. The loss of collateral circulation and vasospasm, or the contraction of blood vessels, add to the problems experienced by the patient. Management usually consists of treating any infection present, reducing pressure, and attempting to provide revascularization.

Appropriate footwear modifications may be very beneficial. For instance, it is possible to use materials and procedures to absorb shock, to accommodate existing deformities, and to make modifications to provide for joint stability. Surgical shoes, extra-depth inlay shoes, reinforced shoe counters, and custom-molded shoes are also useful. Special lasts, Velcro closures, sole wedges for stabilization, heel elevations, metatarsal rocker bars, soft uppers, and cushion soles are only a few of the modifications that can be made to footwear to minimize the effects of decreased arterial blood flow.

Disease of the neurological system may also affect the foot and thus ambulation. Cerebrovascular accidents, Parkinson's disease, and peripheral neuropathies (changes in nerve conduction) are examples of conditions that may limit ambulation by producing deformities and keratotic lesions. The key again is early and continuing management and careful follow-up. To some degree, management has been classed as "routine foot care" and is covered by Medicare *only* when there is an associated risk. With noncoverage comes patient neglect and the development of complications, which are then covered but are more expensive.

Emotional Manifestations

Foot problems may be a manifestation of emotional illness in some patients. Psychological problems can manifest in the foot as hysterical paralysis, nervous tremors, inflammation of the skin as a result of nervous scratching, excessive sweating, and itching. Clearly, many diseases affecting the foot, such as gout and diabetes mellitus, may be complicated by secondary emotional difficulties.

When the symptoms do not match the clinical findings, a foot problem may represent a cry for help. The foot, foot pain, and limitations in ambulation may be an expression of deeper problems, particularly in the elderly mentally ill or retarded. Thus, the neglect of common foot problems in the elderly in mental health programs usually results in decreased ambulation, which encourages institutionalization.

Conclusion

In its final report, the 1981 White House Conference on Aging stated the following:

> Recommendation Number 148:
>
> Comprehensive foot care be provided for the elderly in a manner equal to care provided for other parts of the human body, to permit patients to remain ambulatory.
>
> Implementation:
>
> Remove current Medicare exclusions which preclude comprehensive foot care.

The ability to remain mobile and active requires appropriate foot health. Keeping patients walking is a goal that needs to be met if the elderly are to maintain a high quality of life. Studies indicate that about 80 percent of all older patients will at some time develop foot problems requiring care. Given this high prevalence of foot problems in older patients, complicated by chronic diseases and mental health problems, addressing foot care needs is essential. Foot health and care should be part of the comprehensive health care for older Americans. Maintaining the ability to be active and ambulatory is one way of ensuring dignity and self-esteem in the elderly.

How You Can Prevent Foot Problems

Foot care for those of you who are older and in the prime of your lives, that is, your golden years, is an essential part of your total health care. Much of the ability to remain active and productive rests with good foot health so that you can continue to walk.

First, you must avoid doing those things that add to the danger of decreasing blood circulation to your feet. Pressure, cold, and smoking generally are harmful because they tend to decrease blood flow. The everyday activities that can produce pressure on blood vessels include sitting with your legs crossed, wearing socks with elastic tops, and wearing round elastic garters. In addition, wading, swimming, or bathing in cold water should be avoided.

The second major area of prevention involves breaks in the skin and infection. Any disruption in the skin surface can produce an infection unless immediate care is taken. You can avoid such breaks from burns, irritations, cuts, and/or other injuries by a variety of methods. For example, do not put your feet in hot water or add hot water to your bath without testing the temperature of the water. Generally, your bath or shower temperature should be between 85 and 90 degrees Fahrenheit. If you do not have a proper thermometer, test the water with your elbow or wrist. Be extremely careful if you use a hot water bottle or heating pad for any reason. It is generally best to avoid their use unless they have been prescribed by your practitioner.

Third, do not use corn plasters or commercial corn or ingrown toenail cures or remedies. These preparations are acid in nature and destroy tissue far beyond their original intent. Once there is tissue loss, breaks in the skin occur; some form of infection usually results. Second-degree chemical burns of the skin are also a common result of using these preparations. Although caution labels that apply to older patients may appear on the package, the printing is usually small and the label difficult to read or even to understand. If you avoid the purchase, you avoid the use.

Other things to avoid to maintain good foot health include sunburn, wearing rundown shoes, wearing worn-out stockings, treating your own foot problems with sharp instruments and digging into the corners of your toenails, and walking barefoot, even at home.

Washing your feet daily and wearing clean stockings or socks are a must. You should inspect your feet at least twice a week and look for such things as redness, blisters, cuts or scratches, or cracks between your toes or on your heels. Any discoloration or other changes should also be noted. As we grow older, there is some loss of sensation in the feet, so that visual examination becomes essential. Help your primary physician and your podiatrist help you by telling them of any changes in your feet and by making yourself a part of your own health-care team. If you do notice some change or abnormality, early reporting and care usually prevent serious trouble. You should remember that all health professionals work together to help keep you healthy and walking.

You should wear shoes that not only fit your feet but fit the occasion. Selecting a shoe is most important. The widest part of the shoe should match the widest part of your foot. The shoe should follow the natural outline of your foot and fit snugly without being tight. If you have an existing deformity, special lasts or shoes may be needed. These include special modifications that compensate for existing deformities and changes that have taken place over the years.

For the most part, shoes for general use should be firm enough to help keep your foot in position in the shoe. The heel should give a wide base of support (about 1¼ inches for women). Athletic shoes are wonderful for the activities they are designed for and should not be purchased by size, but by fit. There should be about three-quarters of an inch of space beyond your longest toe (usually the big toe), when you stand. The toe box, or toe cap, should be round and high to allow space for your toes. The shoe upper should be soft and flexible. The lining should be smooth and free of ridges and wrinkles. Buy shoes toward the end of the day to allow for any swelling that may occur as the day goes on. Wear new shoes for gradually extended short periods of time until you are used to the change.

The use of a water-washable cream at night will help to keep your skin soft; dry skin may lead to cracking. The use of a foot powder will also help to keep your feet dry and to prevent friction.

The purpose of this brief section is to help you understand why your feet need special care and how to prevent foot problems. The next job is up to you. Only you can try to remember and follow these simple rules—and thus prevent the serious trouble you could have. I sincerely hope you do.

B. The Foot Heart, the Foot, and the Joys of Walking

CHARLES R. BRANTINGHAM, D.P.M.

Foot and ankle movement have a vital effect, little understood by most people, on the circulation of blood through the body. Heart action and gravity pump blood into the lower extremities, where it tends to become pooled. Blood pressure in the upright human does not get the blood back to the heart.

Rather, the return of blood to the heart and to the brain is the function of valves in the veins and the action of the muscles.

All of the muscles below the knee are foot muscles, and 70 to 80 percent of the valves in the veins are in this region. The valves are arranged so that they will allow blood to flow only toward the heart. Because this structure, variously called the *venous pump,* the *muscles pump,* or the *peripheral venous heart,* acts as a second heart, we call it the *foot heart*.

The importance of the foot heart is illustrated by the following example. If you were tied to a tree, fifteen minutes after you stopped struggling you would black out and your head would fall forward. About twenty minutes later, there would be brain damage. And forty to sixty minutes later, you would be dead. This happens because, when a person stands perfectly still or remains upright without moving, so much blood is pumped into the lower extremities, where, without foot movement, blood stasis occurs, that legs swell and 15 to 20 percent of the blood is lost to blood flow in the body. During the time of the Roman Empire, people were often put to death this way, by being tied to a cross in an upright position.

The foot heart controls the volume of blood flow from the right side of the heart and regulates cardiac output. The adequate function of this structure tends to prevent the development of varicose veins and helps circulation, both of which can be problems for the elderly. This explanation points up the profound importance of foot movement and the value of walking activities.

The structure of the foot, with its rounded bones in the heel and the ball, is best suited to function on the natural terrain of the earth, pathways, trails, and meadows. Yet, we smooth out our earth by turning paths into sidewalks and placing our shopping areas in malls with terrazzo floors. We walk on surfaces really designed for the wheel. The sidewalk of today has just been a secondary structure that gets the pedestrian out of the way of the car.

The foot is tough and will take more abuse than any other part of the body, and it will try to adjust to that abuse. But the constant battering finally results in foot problems. Only people with short, stubby feet and short toes are really comfortable living on flat surfaces.

If you live in such a way that you get the kinds of pressure on your feet that you would get on hillsides, in meadows, and on pathways, your foot will retain its integrity; it will not develop the problems that we see and treat in urban living.

When you walk on varied surfaces, the muscles of the foot get more exercise, which causes a squeezing action that pumps blood back to the heart and enhances circulation. If you want to test this, try standing rigidly in one place without moving your toes for fifteen minutes. You'll probably pass out. Blood is not being circulated back up into your brain. (During World War II, I counseled military personnel to wiggle their toes while standing at attention.)

Because the human being has not evolved to the point of having wheels instead of feet, it is much better for your health to walk on varied terrain. When you walk, stray onto the grass of the parkway for a few paces, or pick a route that is partly uphill or downhill. Any variation in the terrain, even though small, feels better and gives some sensory stimuli to the body. These feelings bring a kind of joy as we walk. The pads that podiatrists have traditionally placed in patients' shoes are really providing artificial terrain that simulates natural terrain.

The criteria for a healthful, comfortable, and safe urban walkway were developed and first studied in shopping centers by doctors functioning under the working name of the "International Academy for Standing and Walking Fitness." These criteria involve changed surfaces in the mall every 120 paces, 80 paces, and 60 paces, from carpet to tile to wood to terrazzo. This variation provides senior citizens, who often walk in the mall, a more healthful surface and, because of increased comfort, encourages additional walking. We have discovered that people stay in such a mall two or three times as long as they stay in one with only a terrazzo floor.

Members of the academy search for places offering healthful and comfortable walking surfaces. They do so in order to honor the business or community offering a varied terrain to workers, customers, or residents. The first mall to be honored was Buena Park Mall in California, for floor surfaces that vary from brick to carpet to wood.

The academy is also anxious to work with cities to improve public walkways in order to encourage more walking. The city of Long Beach, California, was the first city to be eligible for the academy's award. It developed a permanent walking path through the downtown shoreline that provides a textured surface through a series of grooves. Santa Barbara also encourages walking. It has marvelous tiled sidewalks in the downtown area. You find yourself wanting to walk.

This structure, the foot heart, vital to the circulation of blood through the body, can be greatly helped by planned walkways in shopping malls. And we are saying to cities (and we hope you will, too), "Revamp your sidewalks, and pattern them for people rather than just for getting people out of the way of vehicles." We all, including and perhaps especially the elderly, will be the better for it.

Suggested Reading

C. R. Brantingham, "Varied Terrain Floor Surface Takes the Load Off Your Feet," *American Pharmacy,* 24:10 (October 1984), p. 658.

C. R. Brantingham, B. E. Beekman, C. N. Moss, and R. B. Gordon, "Enhanced Venous Pump Activity as a Result of Standing on a Varied Terrain Floor Surface," *Journal of Occupational Medicine,* 12 (1970), pp. 164–169.

C. R. Brantingham, B. E. Beekman, C. N. Moss, and R. B. Gordon, *Stress Reducing Floor Surface System at Standing Work Places and Walkways,* presented at the International Academy for Standing and Walking Fitness meeting in conjunction with the International Congress on Podology, Copenhagen, Denmark, May 6–10, 1982.

Arthur E. Helfand, *Clinical Podogeriatrics.* Baltimore: Williams & Wilkins, 1981.

Arthur E. Helfand, *Public Health and Podiatric Medicine.* Baltimore: Williams & Wilkins, 1987.

Arthur E. Helfand, "Putting Some Life Back into Living," *Focus on Geriatric Care and Rehabilitation.* Frederick, MD: Aspen Publications, 1989.

5

A Review of Nonpathological and Pathological Changes in the Aging Eye

William M. Ludlam, O.D., F.A.A.O. and
Allan N. Freid, O.D., F.A.A.O.

Introduction

Vision care is the second largest national *unmet* health-care need of the elderly, after dental care. The following are some important statistics that underlie this claim:

- Of the visually impaired in the United States in 1985, 70 percent were sixty-five years of age and older. A visually impaired person is either partially sighted or functionally blind. *Partially sighted* means that, even with correction, the corrected visual acuity of the better eye does not exceed 20/70; that is, a partially sighed person can see at 20 feet what person with a 20/20 correction can see at 70 feet. A person who is functionally blind is either totally blind or can, at most, see some light.
- Of those over sixty-five years old 17 percent were functionally blind or partially sighted.
- In 1986, 52 percent of the legally blind in the United States were 65 and older. *Legally blind* means that the best cor-

rected visual acuity in the better eye does not exceed 20/200.

- One study noted that as many as 77 percent of the legally blind had some recorded form vision on an acuity chart or a Snellen chart (commonly used for vision testing). Hence, the major portion even of those classified as blind should be treated clinically as partially sighted.
- A 1973 study estimated partially sighted in the United States at 6 million, including 1.3 million functioning as legally blind.

As is apparent from the foregoing, the elderly suffer disproportionately from visual problems. The changes in visual function in the aging eye are brought about by a combination of optical, physiological, and pathological factors. In this chapter, we will discuss in some detail how these changes affect each anatomical component of the eye (see Figure 1).

Eyelids

The actual eye opening may be reduced because of flaccid lids, enophthalmos (a retraction of the eyeball into the orbit), and weakening of the levator muscle that controls the raising of the upper lid. These conditions often reduce the level of light entering the eye and cause the lashes to obstruct the pupils, making the upward gaze somewhat more difficult.

As the lids become thinner and more flaccid, a "saggy" and "baggy" appearance results. This has a cosmetic effect as well as contributing to the above-mentioned physiological problems.

Xanthelasma, a fatty deposit on the upper lids, sometimes further adds to the tendency of the upper lids to droop. Although surgical removal may provide temporary relief, the deposits usually return within months.

Eyelashes and, to a lesser extent, eyebrows tend to retain their pigmentation despite a generalized depigmentation of the hair covering the head and the body.

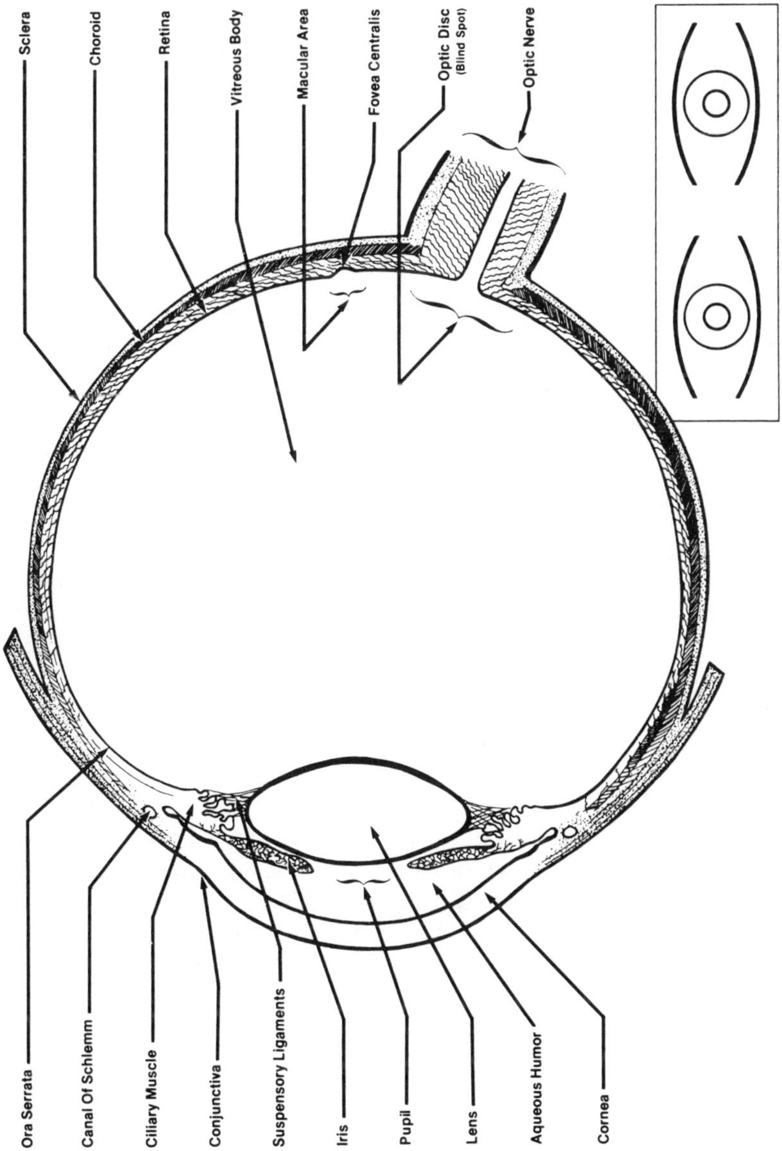

Figure 1. Schematic section of the human eye. Courtesy of the American Optometric Association.

Entropion (a turning inward of the lower lid margin) and trichiasis (in which the lashes scratch the cornea) also increase in occurrence.

Lacrimal Apparatus

Tearing generally decreases with age. This decrease in lacrimation is thought to be due to an increase in connective tissue in the lacrimal gland that supplants the tear-producing tissue. The reduction in lacrimation is generally 50 percent between adolescence and the age of sixty-five.

The ratio of the various elements making up the composition of tears also changes with age. A reduction in the amount of oil results in a more watery composition, faster evaporation, and tears spilling over the lid. This condition may, in fact, afford less protection and lubrication for the cornea.

Serious dry eye from reduction to tear flow can cause corneal damage. With failure to keep the cornea moist, scarring and infection occur, which, in turn, can result in blindness. This condition requires long-term supportive treatment, such as the use of artificial tears, ocular ointments, and/or taping the lids shut while sleeping.

Apposition disorders (failure of the lids to close during blink or while sleeping), caused by alteration of the fit of the lid on the cornea and the conjunctiva, produce changes in the lid–bulbar interface and interfere with the formation of the lacrimal lake (the stream of collected tears) along the margin of the lower lid. Ectropion, in which the lid stretches and becomes more flaccid so that the lid falls away and loses contact with the eyeball and the space fills with tears, and entropion, in which the margin of the lid turns in toward the eyeball, scratches the cornea, and also does not transport the tears toward the punctum at the nasal corner of the lid, resulting in dry eye, are two of the most common apposition disorders. The puncta, or hole in the nasal corner of the lid that drains excess tears, and drainage mechanisms into the nasal lining are thus not able to properly drain the tears, and constant epiphora (tears draining down the cheek) results. This condition puts the eye, the drainage system, and the surrounding skin at risk of the development of infection.

Lysozyme, an enzyme in tear fluid that is a powerful antibacterial and antifungal agent that helps prevent eye infections, does not lessen with age; other factors tend to dilute the eye's antibacterial defenses. The reduction of lacrimal flow and the increased addition of external lubricants, such as eye drops or salves, make the eyes more vulnerable to invading infectious agents.

Lagophthalmos is a condition in which the eyelids never fully close during blinking; in the nocturnal variety, the lids are at least partially open during sleep. This condition causes tear evaporation, ocular dryness, and a reduction in the content of lysozyme and lactoferrin, two of the most powerful antibacterial agents known to science. Consequently, the opportunity for corneal and conjunctival infection and discomfort increases.

Conjunctiva and Sclera

The conjunctiva, or mucous membrane and layer of collapsed blood vessels lining the eyelid and part of the eyeball, assumes a more yellow appearance as a result of fat deposits in the subconjunctival layers. The tissue also undergoes changes, thickening and losing its elasticity. There is a 40 percent decrease in splitting strength (the force needed to split or crack conjunctival tissue) of the conjunctiva between the ages of thirty and sixty. This decrease causes more frequent tearing from trauma and pressure, as in coughing and sneezing, and leads to an increased occurrence of subconjunctival hemorrhages.

Conjunctivitis, or inflammation of the conjunctiva, is seen commonly in the elderly. It may be caused by viral, allergic, bacterial, or environmental factors. Management depends on the identification of the underlying cause and the institution of the proper therapy. Conjunctivitis is generally not sight-threatening unless there is involvement of the cornea. Smears and cultures should be obtained to better aid in diagnosis and subsequent therapy.

The aging sclera—the thick, white, fibrous outer coat enclosing the eyeball—also assumes a yellowish tint. This condition, caused by lipid deposits primarily on the front portion of the sclera, is usually not sight-threatening.

Scleral rigidity increases, and the scleral vascular system undergoes tortuous alterations that become more extreme in the presence of generalized arteriosclerosis. Scleral rigidity affects intraocular pressure, increasing the damage to retinal nerves in glaucoma, a condition of increased pressure in the eyeball.

Cornea

Changes in the composition and the refractive index (the amount that light is bent or refracted by a tissue) of the precorneal film and the cornea reduce the "luster" of the aging eye. This is only a cosmetic problem.

Changes in corneal curvature contribute to astigmatism. The cornea is normally spherical. In the younger person, pressure from the upper and lower eyelids sometimes pushes the cornea into a horizontal football shape, causing "with-the-rule" astigmatism. As a person ages, increasing lid flaccidity reduces lid pressure, allowing the cornea to assume a vertical football shape. This is "against-the-rule" astigmatism.

Sometimes, a white ring, called the *arcus senilis*, is formed when fat invades the corneal margin. Although it causes no known primary visual changes, there is a disturbing cosmetic alteration in appearance. The presence of the ring may also indicate faulty metabolism of cholesterol and other fats, which should be considered in overall health evaluations.

A major age-related alteration in the cornea is the decline in the number of endothelial cells, the cells that line the inside surface of the cornea. The endothelium acts as a pump to keep excess water out of the cornea, keeping it transparent and the surfaces regular. One study shows a reduction in the average number of cells in the single-layered endothelium from 3,200 at age twenty to 2,500 in the typical seventy-five-year-old. Once a critical number of these irreplaceable cells is lost (1,500 is thought to be that level), the endothelial barrier function is diminished, and as a result, corneal edema, or swelling from water inflow, occurs. In severe cases, this edema leads to decreased acuity, halos around lights, pain, and bullous keratopathy, a severe disease of the cornea that can lead to blindness.

Pigmentary deposits on the rear surface of the cornea also increase in frequency with age. Although usually not threatening to vision, these deposits reduce the amount of light reaching the retina.

Iris and Pupil

A reduction in the size of the pupil, called *miosis,* is one of the most readily noticeable changes in aging. It is caused by the same decrease in the sympathetic tone of the autonomic nervous system that causes enophthalmos, or retraction of the eyeball. Miosis has several effects on vision, not all of them disadvantageous. Less illumination enters the eye, but there is a greater depth of field. That is, a smaller (or miotic) pupil causes a more extended clear field of vision without refocusing. This is an advantage for older people, who lose the ability to change focus with increasing age. Also, with miosis, there is a reduction of the effect on acuity of aberrations (e.g., distortion and curvature of field) and ametropia (optical errors of the eye corrected by spectacles).

Some depigmentation of the iris occurs. In lightly pigmented eyes (gray and blue), the iris sphincter becomes more visible. The iris sphincter is a circular muscle surrounding the pupil that makes the pupil opening larger and smaller in response to light level, fear, or focusing effort. The pigment fragments from the iris deposit on the rear surface of the cornea and the front surface of the crystalline lens, float in the aqueous humor, and flow into the spaces of the trabeculae in the filtration angle. This factor may be partially responsible for the increased incidence of glaucoma in the elderly.

Crystalline Lens

Cataract constitutes the most frequently observed alteration of the crystalline lens in the aging eye. *Cataract* is defined as a reduction of the clarity of the material of which the lens is composed. It has been estimated that 65 percent of the "normal" population between fifty-one and sixty years old has "senile" cataract to some extent, and this percentage rises to 95 percent over the age of sixty-one. Surgical removal of the cataractous lens remains the treatment of choice, and a plastic implant lens is used to replace the removed lens.

The lens continues to grow throughout life. Its mass triples on average from 80 milligrams at birth to 240 milligrams at age seventy. The volume increases at a slightly lower rate than does the mass because, with the ongoing growth of the lens, there is a slight but continuous increase in the density due to the compression of the lens fibers in the nuclear region. Although the hair and nails also continue to grow throughout life, the lens is unique in that the new cells do not replace preexisting ones but add to those in place. Thus, at any one time, the crystalline lens is composed of the full complement of all the cells it has ever contained. Over time, it becomes less flexible and becomes unable to change shape to allow clear focus for reading and close work, so that "reading" or near-work corrective lenses are required.

Optically, the lens both transmits light and refracts, or bends, it. As people age, variations in the lens's transmitting properties affect both the amount and the spectral distribution of the light reaching the retina. The lens usually yellows with age (the older, the yellower) so that it is more difficult for the elderly observer to see violet and deep blue because of the lens's filtering action.

The new cells in the lens are added primarily to the front and equatorial portions. This process produces a tendency toward flattening of the anterior lens surface, which is thought to be the major reason for the increase in hyperopia (farsightedness) of the aging refractive system. There also occurs an increase in axial thickness of the lens, with a concomitant reduction in the depth of the anterior chamber. This process causes increased pressure in the eye, which increasingly predisposes the aging eye to closed-angle glaucoma.

The mechanism whereby the lens changes focus for different distances is called *accommodation*. The reduction in the lens's ability to accommodate is a lifelong process, but it becomes critical in the decade of the forties and later, when adequate focus cannot be accomplished or maintained at the habitual near-working or reading distance. This condition, termed *presbyopia* (old sight), has three causes: an increase in the viscosity of the lens material; an increase in the overall size of the lens, which makes it less manageable by the ciliary muscle; and a decrease in the strength of the ciliary muscle. The ciliary muscle is at the equator of the lens and changes the shape of the lens for different focusing distances.

These factors, which reduce the flexibility of focus of the aging eye, necessitate, almost universally, the use of multifocal spectacle lenses (bifocals and trifocals) by the elderly.

Vitreous Body

The vitreous body is the viscous, clear material that fills the posterior half of the eye. Located behind the crystalline lens, it helps the eyeball keep its shape. There is still disagreement about what constitutes normal physiological change and what constitutes pathological change in the aging vitreous. These disagreements are due, in turn, to differences about the basic nature of the vitreous: Is it a sol (a thick solution or colloidal suspension) or a gel? Is it an organized tissue to begin with?

Although the shrinking of the vitreous is a normal process, its causes remain unclear. Is it due to senile dehydration, a loss of both extracellular and intracellular water? This is a general characteristic in all aging tissues. Or is the shrinking caused by vitreous liquefaction, in which intracellular water does not appear to change, but extracellular water increases. A third school holds that both of these factors occur simultaneously and that liquefaction occurs in the inner vitreous while dehydration occurs in the outer, surface segment.

In most people in their fifties and sixties, some vitreous detachment (separation of the vitreous from the retina) is believed to occur between the firm attachments at the optic nerve head at the back of the eye and the ora serrata, the extreme forward edge of the retina. One study concluded that 65 percent of the population have vitreous detachment by age seventy. Vitreous detachments are not sight-threatening. They must be differentiated from retinal detachments, which are always serious. The only visual disturbances that accompany vitreous detachment are flashes of light that start in the upper retina and over months, sometimes years, proceed to central and finally lower levels of the retina. The person perceives these flashes in the opposite field; that is, the upper level flashes are seen below eye level, the central ones are seen at central level, and the lower level flashes, in the later stages of vitreous detachment, are seen above eye level. There is also a report of many dusty particles, or specks of pigment called *pepper,* floating in the vitreous, which are absorbed and disappear over time.

A second change in the vitreous associated with aging is synchesis scintillans, a condition of cholesterol deposits in the vitreous. When the eye is moved rapidly up and down, these deposits appear to cascade down like a waterfall. This effect creates only minor visual disturbances when the deposits pass quickly through the line of sight. The condition almost always occurs in both eyes and is observed mostly in people in their seventies and eighties. It is believed to be associated with faulty lipid metabolism.

Asteroid hyalosis is a third vitreous condition occurring in the elderly, in which the stearins and lecithin, fatty substances usually found in the blood, leak out of the walls of the retinal blood vessels and into the vitreous. These deposits are essentially stationary in the vitreous and usually occur in each eye. They produce only mild visual disturbances, the principal one being a need for more light in viewing tasks involving fine detail.

Retina and Fundus

The scientific literature shows that the retina is relatively free of nonpathological changes as people age. Although some cell loss occurs in the retina, as it does in many structures in the human central nervous system, the changes in the retina and its neural connections that accompany normal aging are largely inferred by patients' behavioral or visual changes rather than by observed structural changes. Most changes in the retinal function of the fundus (the rear of the eye constituting the retina, the optic nerve, and blood vessels) with aging are due to changes in its vascular supply. Thus, the changes in the fundus observable with the ophthalmoscope are mostly confined to the appearance of the retinal vessels and the underlying choroid, the layer of blood vessels immediately behind the retina that supplies it with nutriment.

With age, the foveal reflex diminishes. The fovea is the small area at the rear of the retina where vision is clearest. The retina, which is ten layers thick over most of its area, reduces to three layers of thickness at the fovea. Thus, a depression, or pit, is formed. When a light from an ophthalmoscope is shone into the eye, this foveal pit produces a bright reflection known as the *foveal reflex*.

Yellowish-white areas often visible in the fundus of the aging eye are attributable to the exposure of Bruch's membrane, a thin layer of transparent tissue that lies between the retina and the vitreous and attaches them. Small secretions called *drusen* frequently appear later in life, increase in number, and sometimes become pigmented. They have been variously described as pathological choroidal lesions by some authors and innocuous secretions of the pigment epithelium (the outermost layer of the retina immediately in front of the choroid) by others. Because the inner layers of the choroid become more visible, a blotchy appearance of the fundus is often noted because of depigmentation of the retinal pigment epithelium.

Age-related macular degeneration is the major dysfunction of the retina in the elderly eye. The macula, which surrounds the fovea, is the area of clearest vision in the retina at the back of the eye. When the fundus is viewed with the ophthalmoscope, the macula is the area free of blood vessels. It receives its blood supply from the choroid. It is thought that, in macular degeneration, this blood supply from the choroid is interfered with and the cone receptors are destroyed by lack of circulation to the macula. This condition accounts for about 30 percent of the patients with reduced acuity in the seventy-five- to eighty-five-year-old category, as compared to 7 percent with glaucoma and 7 percent with general retinal pathology. The average age of onset of macular degeneration is sixty-five years, and the other eye becomes involved usually within four years.

Although the disease is mainly associated with aging, the reduction in central acuity probably has multiple causes. Such factors may include detachment of the pigment epithelium, atrophy of the pigment epithelium, and thinning of the retina resulting in a macular hole, with secondary changes in Bruch's membrane associated with drusen and irregular pigment changes. The current therapy for the condition centers on the laser treatment of leaking vessels sufficiently distant from the fovea. Refractive correction should not be overlooked in clinical treatment, as well as low-vision aids such as telescopic or microscopic spectacles, which enhance vision for people who, through disease or accident, have reduced vision.

Visual Fields

The size of the visual field as measured under prescribed conditions generally decreases with age. Thus, the extent of the field measured with a 1-millimeter white target at 1 meter at sixty years of age is smaller than that of the average, normal twenty-year-old, even if pupil size is controlled. This decrease does not necessarily mean a decrease in neural function. For example, as the crystalline lens becomes more opaque, it causes a reduction in the light reaching the retina, which then decreases the extent of the field. Clinically, the presence of scotomas, or local areas of reduced sensitivity in the visual field, as well as sudden changes has greater importance than a slightly reduced field. The regular measurement of visual fields in elderly patients is recommended as a means of monitoring ocular health and physiology.

Oculomotor System

The oculomotor system, which consists of six muscles on the outside of each eye, controls the function of the eye muscles that move the eye. Irregularities in the system result either from slow changes in oculomotor balance (the alignment of the eyes) due to accommodative or accommodative-convergence changes, or from a sudden change often associated with systemic or central nervous system pathology. The condition becomes critical when the patient loses voluntary control of binocular alignment, or the ability to coordinate both eyes in aiming and focusing. The condition in which the eyes are not aligned is called *strabismus* and is usually accompanied by diplopia, or double vision. When the onset of this condition is sudden, the strabismus deviation, or the angle of eye turn, varies according to the different directions of the gaze. In this instance, the possibility of active pathology should be carefully explored. Some possible causes of binocular pathology include diabetes, thyroid gland dysfunction, trauma, and hypertension.

Ocular palsy (the partial paralysis of one or more of the eye muscles) is found in many patients with diabetes. It often affects the third cranial nerve and may include pupil abnormalities as well. In older patients, the onset is often gradual. Other symptoms of diabetes also include headaches, increased thirst and urination, overweight, constipation, and increased appetite with loss of weight.

Thyrotoxicosis, or thyroid gland dysfunction, is often accompanied by exophthalmos, or abnormal protrusion of the eyeball, and may feature muscle palsy as well. Interest in this condition has been brought before the public lately because of the media coverage of the condition in President and Mrs. Bush. In addition to vertical diplopia, the symptoms may include retraction of the upper lid, infrequent blinking, and conjunctival infection.

Head injuries (traumas) caused by falls, blows to the head, automobile accidents, and so on often result in esotropia (crossed eye). This condition is related to an injury to the sixth cranial nerve, which has a long, very exposed course in the skull.

High blood pressure increase is a cause of oculomotor paresis (partial paralysis) with increasing age. Hypertension is estimated to be a causative factor in about 10 percent of the muscle palsies found in older patients. The general symptoms of high blood pressure include dizziness, breathlessness, ringing in the ears, and headache.

If one is to treat oculomotor anomalies, the underlying cause must first be identified and treated. The visual disturbances can be treated as deemed appropriate with a prism in the spectacle lens, vision training, alteration of the head position, or, in extreme cases, the occlusion of one eye.

Presbyopia, if it becomes very severe, may also result in binocular disturbances that may require changes in bifocals and the use of a prism to increase fusion ability. Vision therapy may also be necessary. Increased exophoria, a tendency for the two eyes to turn outward, with the resulting fusional deficits, may cause intermittent double vision.

Summary and Conclusion

It can be seen that both normal and pathological changes occur in the aging eye.

Changes in the lids and the lacrimal system mostly cause small inconsequential changes in vision and eye function. Ectropion (in which the lid pulls away from the eyeball) may cause epiphora (tears constantly running down the cheeks) with excoriation of the skin at the corners of the eye. Entropion (the turning inward of the lower lid margin) may be more serious if the inwardly turned lashes cause abrasion of the cornea, which may lead to scarring, discomfort, and danger of corneal infection. Severe dry eye in xerophthalmia (reduction of tear flow) may lead to scarring and visual loss as well as marked discomfort.

Corneal and conjunctival changes also produce minor visual dysfunction, except in cases of corneal ulceration and dystrophy. Corneal shape alterations may result in astigmatic changes that can be corrected with spectacles or contact lenses.

Iris and pupil changes cause minor changes in vision. Pupillary miosis, or contraction, causes a reduction in the amount of light entering the eye but reduces the effect of optical errors and increases depth of field. Depigmentation of the iris increases free-floating pigment, which deposits on the front lens surface and/or the rear surface of the cornea and tends to clog the filtration angle and raise the possibility of closed-angle glaucoma.

The crystalline lens tends toward opacity with age, which causes cataract, with diminished acuity and altered color vision. Surgical removal of the lens and its replacement with an implanted plastic lens is the treatment of choice at present. Spectacle correction for both distant and near vision can then be applied with a multifocal lens (bifocal, progressive addition lens, or trifocal).

Oculomotor changes that cause double vision and limitation of gaze may indicate severe central nervous system dysfunction from stroke, trauma, or disease, such as diabetes or thyrotoxicosis. Double vision may also accompany refractive and accommodative changes with aging and can be corrected with lenses or vision therapy.

Normal vitreous changes are generally not sight-threatening, but vitreous detachment must be carefully differentiated from retinal detachment, which is sight-threatening.

Retinal changes include a normal decrease of retinal receptors with aging, as well as a small diminution in central visual acuity and the extent of the visual field. Systemic and ocular vascular changes affect choroidal and macular metabolism and may seriously affect central and peripheral visual sensitivity. The latter occurs with macular degeneration. Elevated intraocular pressure in glaucoma also affects peripheral visual function initially, and if uncontrolled, it will usually eventually result in painful blindness. Macular degeneration and diabetic retinopathy (disease of the retina) constitute the largest causes of legal blindness in the United States.

In combination, the two eye-care professions, optometry and ophthalmology, have their unique missions in eye care to prevent, correct, and ameliorate the various conditions enumerated and described above. Harmoniously working together toward this end, both can well serve the aging population. Because visual care is still the second largest national unmet health-care need, it is apparent that this task has not been accomplished. Better interprofessional cooperation and enhanced societal awareness are essential if we are to change this situation.

Suggested Reading

E. Mehr and A. Freid, *Low Vision Care* (2nd ed.). New York: Professional Press, 1989.

A. Rosenbloom and M. Morgan (eds.), *Vision and Aging: General and Clinical Perspectives.* New York: Professional Press, 1986.

R. Sekuler, D. Kline, and K. Dismukes, *Aging and Human Visual Function.* New York: Alan R. Liss, 1982.

6

Chemical Dependency among Older Americans

NICHOLAS A. CUMMINGS, PH.D., LITT.D.

Introduction

Our generation now comprises 11 percent of the American population. We are a resilient generation, having survived our nation's worst depression, greatest war, and highest inflation. Those in our cohort who were alcoholics, drug addicts, criminals, and otherwise self-destructive have long ago done themselves in. Those of us who have earned the title "senior citizen" are, indeed, survivors. We vote, pay our taxes, worship, support our government, and indulge our grandchildren. Chemical dependency among this remarkable generation seems absurd. Can it be possible? The answer is yes, and we and our children, who are also concerned about us, need to be alerted.

Until recently, the extent of chemical dependency among older Americans was masked by a number of factors. Principal among these is that we are a proud generation, and in contrast to succeeding generations, we are private and do not "let it all hang out." We still respect the doctor and would be ashamed to admit to a drinking or other chemical dependency. We are even ashamed to admit it to ourselves, and we find ways of rationalizing or otherwise avoiding facing the problem. Furthermore, alcohol, pain killers, sleeping pills, antidepressives, and tranquilizers have the propensity in the elderly of markedly increasing their memory deficit. If we are overly using these chemicals, we may simply not remember just how much we drank or how many pills we have taken.

Iatrogenic Chemical Dependency

Much of the chemical dependency among older Americans is iatrogenic, or doctor-induced. No one can say exactly how much, but it is an enormous amount. We are used to younger people looking right through us, but we expect the doctor, whom we respect, to understand us. Many physicians do not. They do not understand that, at any given time, some muscle or some bone in our bodies is always hurting. They do not comprehend that we may be lonely or bored or may feel unwanted by society. So they patronize us ("There, there. You are not as young as you used to be, and you've got to take it easier"), and they give us pills. The elderly are the most overmedicated segment of our society. And if you are a woman as well as elderly, the chances of your being given pills is twice as great.

Because we respect the doctor, we dutifully take the medication as prescribed. Many medications that are safe in younger persons may have severe untoward effects in older patients. The medical profession is always discovering new side effects of medicines. Even something as supposedly safe as aspirin may bring surprises. After aspirin had been in wide use for more than sixty years, it was only recently discovered that aspirin has caused severe, permanent brain damage in some children. The side effects of most medications have not been extensively tested in the elderly. And *combinations* of various medications are little, if at all, understood. Because specialists often prescribe for you without finding out what other, and possibly incompatible, medications you are taking, you are facing "medical roulette."

When medications, or combinations of medications, have a

negative effect, you may suffer memory loss, and because you cannot remember, you may not know your memory has been adversely affected. Another common drug side effect in the elderly is confusion. Because you are confused, you may not know you are confused. I have evaluated patients who were misdiagnosed as suffering from Alzheimer's disease or senile dementia who, once taken off the offending medications, cleared to normal mentation within two weeks. And I have seen patients who were taking more than two dozen different medicines, many of which were questionable if not incompatible, given by a number of different physicians, who were dutifully taking all of these drugs because they respected and believed in their doctors, and they continued the regimen in spite of increasing negative side effects.

Many of us reach our senior years iatrogenically addicted because our physicians have been prescribing sleeping pills, tranquilizers, or pain medication for years. This is even more probable if you are an elderly woman, as many physicians seem to lack patience with what they erroneously regard as the emotional lability of females. These medications are wonder drugs in acute situations. They were not intended to be given over decades. Some of them, such as the benzodiazapines (Librium, Dalmane, Valium, and possibly such more recent cousins as Buspar and Xanax) can, with long use, cause tardive dyskinesias in our older years. A major aspect of this condition is uncontrollable shaking, which can be eliminated only by increasing the dosage of the very medication that brought about the condition in the first place. Soon, the shaking reappears, and the medication has to be increased again, and then again, and again. The result is a zombielike elderly person not unlike most of the residents of our nursing homes.

Any mind-altering medication seems to have an increasingly deleterious effect on the minds of older persons. Something that has been taken for years without side effects to aid in sleep or to tranquilize nervousness may in later years cause exaggerated memory loss, confusion, or dyskinesias. And because the addiction has existed for years, the person is highly resistive to giving it up. Those who have undergone withdrawal through the aid of biofeedback and other nondrug techniques report a significantly improved quality of life. But most elderly addicted persons seem to continue their pattern into eventual mental confusion.

The Elderly and Alcohol

Before we wrongfully conclude that all chemical dependency problems in older Americans are iatrogenic, let us look again, especially at alcohol, which is the most widely abused drug in America today. There are alcohol problems among the elderly, and those studies that show a reduction in the consumption of alcohol by older Americans have not taken into account two factors: (1) chronic alcoholics' mortality rate prevents their reaching advanced years, and (2) many elderly reduce their consumption of alcohol because of illnesses or because they cannot afford it on a reduced income. A significant number of older Americans increase their consumption of alcohol for reasons we shall discuss below.

The majority of older Americans maintain the same level of alcohol consumption that has been characteristic throughout their adult lives. But even this level results in problems. First, the aging process, both physically and mentally, may dramatically reduce the tolerance of alcohol. This means that the same amount of alcohol can now result in levels of intoxication, confusion, or memory loss that did not exist in one's younger years. Various illnesses may even further complicate and reduce alcohol tolerance. Older Americans must be cognizant of these factors and must adjust their drinking patterns as, one hopes, they have adjusted their eating patterns to accommodate the aging process.

Another contributor to alcohol problems in the older American who maintains the same lifelong moderate level of drinking is the medication the person is now taking. Alcohol has a synergistic effect with many medications, greatly increasing the negative side effects. Some medications taken with alcohol may even cause death. Depending on the medicine taken, the older patient must reduce or eliminate alcohol consumption to prevent these side effects. It is our responsibility to ask our doctors whether the prescribed medication is compatible with even a little alcohol. And the problem is further exacerbated in the elderly. Many medications that a younger person can combine with alcohol safely, may lead, in combination with alcohol, to confusion and increased memory loss in the elderly. From years of treating the elderly in these untoward reactions, my own advice to older Americans who are taking any kind of mind-altering drug is not to drink at all.

A significant number of older Americans increase their consumption of alcohol and contribute to a high rate of alcoholism, as evidenced by studies of hospital admissions. The age group sixty-five and older has the highest proportion (approximately 60 percent) of alcohol-related hospital diagnoses that are not primary diagnoses. This means that physicians tend to miss evidences of alcoholism in this age group until these patients are hospitalized for other health reasons, when the alcoholism and its contributions to the patient's overall ill health are identified. It is unfortunate that considerable alcohol-related morbidity in our older population goes undetected and untreated until the ravages of alcoholism become obvious.

A late onset of heavy drinking may begin in response to stressful life experiences, which may include bereavement, economic changes, poor health, or even retirement. The late onset of heavy drinking is most frequent among older Americans of higher socioeconomic status, a fact indicating that the ability to afford alcoholic beverages is a factor.

There are persons who have kept their amount of drinking in check because they had to meet a work schedule. On retiring, this impediment to drinking is removed, and consumption increases. At the extreme end is a retired person who lives alone, has no friends, and does not drive an automobile. His or her heavy drinking may go unhampered and undetected until the tertiary stage. But the boredom and loneliness or the feeling of being not needed that may accompany retirement are enough to increase the alcohol consumption even of those who have not had a history of marginally heavy drinking. Retirement counseling has been demonstrated to reduce alcohol morbidity in our older population, but unfortunately, it is not used as much as it should be.

Ill health may lead to depression, which, in turn, may lead to late-onset heavy drinking. For example, alcohol may lower the perception of pain in severe arthritis and may also numb the depression that often accompanies the condition. Again, counseling that helps the patient to manage physical illness and that treats the depression has been shown to significantly reduce alcohol morbidity among older Americans.

A frequent cause of late-onset drinking is bereavement. The sadness, sense of loss, and loneliness that accompany widowhood render the surviving spouse more prone to attempt to avoid these intense feelings through heavy drinking. The widow or widower of an alcoholic who suddenly begins heavy drinking for the first time on the death of the spouse is well known among psychotherapists. The reason appears to be that the widowed "enabler," now deprived of an alcoholic to enable, becomes the drinker. Recent advances in bereavement counseling indicate that such counseling not only reduces alcohol morbidity but also reduces the abnormally high incidence of cancer and heart disease in the surviving spouse during the first year.

Pain and Chemical Dependency

No discussion of chemical dependency in our older population would be complete without addressing medication for the terminally ill who are in intense pain. For many, laypersons and physicians alike, such medication raises ethical questions. Surveys have indicated that most Americans are in favor of unlimited pain medication for those in severe pain and on the verge of dying. The problem arises in treating those elderly who are in intense pain and whose death is prolonged, not just for months but often for years. Heavy and prolonged doses of medication may not only increase memory deficit and confusion but almost always render people shadows of themselves. This loss of identity may lower the individual's quality of life and restrict relatedness and interaction with loved ones. As tolerance of the medication builds up over months and years, the individual is more and more intellectually and emotionally out of it as he or she becomes increasingly unable to function without larger and larger doses.

If there were no alternatives, this overmedication would be the price for freedom from pain of the patient whose dying is prolonged. Since the early 1980s, impressive gains have been made in the nonpharmacological management of chronic pain. Unfortunately, physicians do not consider this as much as they could, as it is easier to reach for the prescription pad. In such instances, the family and loved ones must become knowledgeable about these alternatives and insist that they be investigated.

Summary

In summary, it can be said that our proud and remarkable generation is not free of chemical dependency problems. Even though most of the chronic alcoholics and drug addicts in our generation have already done themselves in, a late onset of heavy drinking may be brought on by the stresses of this advanced period of life. In addition, the aging process renders us less tolerant of alcohol, and this lessened tolerance may be further complicated by illness and medication. Counseling is an important alternative to the overmedication of older Americans. Although we are the generation that still respects and dutifully obeys the doctor, we can take a cue from our children, who say that health is each person's responsibility, that health education and enlightenment are a must, and that second medical opinions are not only appropriate but often necessary.

Suggested Reading

R. M. Atkinson, "Alcoholism in the elderly population," *Mayo Clinic Procedures*, 63 (1988), pp. 825–828.

G. Maddox, L. N. Robins, and N. Rosenberg (eds.), *Nature and Extent of Alcohol Problems among the Elderly,* Monograph No. 14, DHHS Publication No. (ADM) 84-1321. Washington, DC: Government Printing Office, 1984.

7

The Role of Nursing in Care of the Elderly

LINDA R. PHILLIPS, PH.D., R.N.

Introduction

Nursing professionals currently provide more health care to the elderly than does any other group of health professionals. Regardless of the area of specialization, virtually all nurses in the United States are involved in gerontological nursing, whether they are working in critical care units, in general medical-surgical units, in ambulatory care units, or in home care. In addition, because of the nature of family relationships in this country, even nurses working in areas that seem remote from gerontology, such as maternity and pediatrics, are quite likely to provide some care to elders while providing care to younger individuals.

As members of the largest of the health professions, nurses potentially have more contact with the elderly than does any other group of health professionals. Because of their many employment settings, nurses daily are the most likely of all health-care providers to encounter elderly people. Also, the nature of nursing practice means that nurses have the most sustained contact with elders in the course of providing care.

Not only are nurses involved in the care of the elderly, but the majority of all care provided to the elderly is nursing care. This care is provided by either nurses or nurse extenders (e.g., nursing assistants, home health aides, and family caregivers). Most of the problems encountered by elderly individuals and their caregivers relate to functional abilities and self-care activities, including managing treatment regimes. Whether the focus of the problem is on maintaining or enhancing existing levels of competence, or on remediating deficits in competence, these particular problems fall squarely within the domain of nursing practice.

A much smaller proportion of the problems encountered by the elderly and their caregivers, outside the realm of self-care, are disease-related and may require hospital care. Here, nurses have important responsibilities on the interdisciplinary teams that design and implement disease-focused health care with and for elders and their families.

It is clear, then, that nurses currently have a significant amount of contact with the elderly and play an important role in providing them primary, secondary, and tertiary health care. The nursing role is both intradisciplinary and interdisciplinary. Yet, although the scope of the nurse role is complex, multifaceted, and broad, that role is often viewed narrowly by nurses, paranursing professionals, and policymakers because of the emphasis in this country on cure and high technology, and because of the low status given to women and "women's work." As a consequence, even though the nursing profession has a great effect on and responsibility for providing health care to elderly clients and their families, nursing often has little authority in developing the broad policies that determine the direction of health care for the elderly.

In this chapter, I discuss the scope of the nursing role in (1) shaping the *processes* of the health care of the elderly; (2) determining the *structure* of the health care of the elderly; and (3) defining the *outcomes* of the health care of the elderly. The purpose of this discussion is to identify the areas in which nurses are best able to assume leadership in policymaking positions and to contribute to decisions about health care policy for the elderly.

The Nursing Role in Shaping Processes

Of the three domains, or facets, identified, the nursing role in the process domain of health care for the elderly seems to be the easiest to identify and has been the most universally acknowledged and used. The reason is partly that both the public and the paranursing professionals recognize that (1) by definition, nursing *is* a process involving interpersonal interactions between a care recipient and a care provider, and (2) the nursing contribution to health outcomes is related as much to the manner in which care is provided as it is to the nature of the actual activities. Therefore, many of the essential parts of this role are obvious to all who carefully observe health care delivery.

The three obvious roles of nursing within the process domain of elder care are (1) the day-to-day management of daily-living, clinical, and behavioral problems; (2) the prevention of premature disability and functional decline; and (3) the promotion of the physical, emotional, and spiritual health of elderly clients.

Although these are the most apparent process roles of nurses and the roles that thousands of nurses perform daily for the elderly in this country, by no means do they comprehensively represent *all* roles in relation to elder health care that are uniquely appropriate to nursing. The identification of these three particular roles, although appropriate and accurate, emphasizes the reactive role of nursing in supporting, delivering, and maintaining health care processes. It does not provide an indication of nursing's proactive role in *shaping* the health care processes of older people. This distinction is important because these three traditional roles of nursing reinforce the view that nursing as a discipline focuses on doing rather than leading and shaping.

The less obvious, proactive roles of nursing in the process domain also need to be recognized. The overriding principles that govern the proactive nursing roles in relationship to the aged can be divided into four categories: (1) individualization; (2) humanization; (3) affirmation; and (4) mediation. In addition, it must be noted that nursing's role involves both "micro" and "macro" elements. At the micro level, the appropriate targets for nursing care of the aged include the client, the client and his or her environment, and the aging family unit. At the macro level, the appropriate targets for nursing care of the aged include the aging local, national, and international community.

Individualization involves adapting self-care and health-care regimens to meet the particular lifestyle and preferences of individual clients. Although all health professionals acknowledge the notion of diversity within the aging population as a theoretical concept, addressing the issue of diversity on a client-by-client basis is a role of nursing. It is also a role in which nurses excel.

At the micro level, examples of individualization include adapting a self-care activity such as bathing to the unique preferences of the individual client or adapting a medication regime to his or her particular lifestyle. Other examples of individualization include altering the home environment so that self-care activities such as bathing will be facilitated; altering institutional policies about self-care activities, such as bathing or sleeping, to meet the lifestyle of a particular resident; and assisting the caregiver to adapt a client's medication regime to meet both the requirements of the medication regime and the caregiver's needs for rest and sleep.

At the macro level, examples include negotiating with community service agencies to create schedules for service delivery that meet the desires of the elderly in the community and presenting testimony before official agencies (e.g., congressional committees) about the impact of federal regulations (e.g., Medicare) on the health and well-being of the elderly in this country.

The concept of humanization emphasizes quality of life over technological advancement and cure. Again, although all health professionals acknowledge the importance of the quality of life of our aging population, nursing's unique role rests in putting humanization into practice for individual clients. Four unique nursing roles distinguish gerontological nursing from other types of nursing practice: (1) taking charge; (2) being with the client; (3) empowering the client to make decisions; and (4) understanding and experiencing with the client the meaning of her or his moment-to-moment existence. All four represent examples of nursing's role in humanization at the micro level.

At the macro level, the appropriate model of health care for the elderly has been a point of discussion in this country for a number of years. It has become increasingly clear that the emphasis on the episodic, disease-focused model has been largely ineffective in meeting the needs of most of the elderly for two reasons. First, the majority of health problems experienced by the elderly involve chronic, ongoing conditions that are manageable, though not resolvable, and involve functional and self-care limitations rather than recovery or precipitous death. Second, the majority of health problems experienced by the elderly are multifaceted and complex, involving physical, emotional, social, economic, cultural, and lifestyle aspects.

For those elders in institutions, it is also becoming increasingly clear that models that emphasize quantity of life over quality of life are not meeting the needs of the majority of the clients. In both settings, the health care model most likely to be effective with aging clients is one that accounts for the complexity of the problems encountered in caring for this age group and draws on a unified rather than a compartmentalized view of the client.

Nursing and the models for nursing practice are based largely on the principles that (1) clients have the right to self-determination and independent decision making; (2) clients are holistic in nature, and their health and well-being are affected by the interaction of physiological, pathological, psychological, social, financial, and environmental factors; and (3) nursing has a role in assisting clients to optimize their health, to improve their quality of life, and to achieve comfort. Nursing, ideally suited to putting this model into practice, has a unique mission in representing this model to the elderly and to the paranursing professionals who provide them care.

The concept of affirmation involves a positive, developmental view of aging and aging clients rather than a view that defines aging in terms of decremental loss. The predominant social, medical, and professional view of aging is that aging is a period of personal decline. As a result, the changes that occur as a result of aging (e.g., changes in the sensory apparatus) are interpreted as evidence that aging is decay and deterioration. Loss and illness are themes that are emphasized in academic and popular descriptions of the aging experience.

For gerontologists in all the health professions, the predominant focus is very different. Forestalling aging as long as possible and erasing the effects of aging from body systems is their goal.

At the micro level, nursing practice is characterized by sustained, physical and emotional, intimate interaction between nurses and clients. The intimacy involved in nursing permits the development of affectional bonds between nurses and clients that make impossible a strict belief in aging as only a period of loss and decline. As a consequence, within nursing, there has developed a "negentropic" view that permits aging and aging clients to be placed within the context of living. According to this view, aging is seen (1) as an essential developmental process that is inevitable and irreversible and (2) as the thread that provides coherence and meaning to life. This view is inherent in the fourth unique role of gerontological nursing: understanding and experiencing the meaning of moment-to-moment existence. Nursing has a unique role in fostering, developing, and promoting this view of aging clients among all those who provide care to the aged.

The concept of mediation drives those nursing roles that involve the coordination of health care services. Case management, continuity of care, discharge planning, and advocacy are as old as nursing practice itself. In the tradition of Lillian Wald, the nurse who founded the internationally known Henry Street Settlement in New York City in 1893 and the world's first public-school nursing system, case management and coordination of health care services have been hallmarks of public health nursing for the past one hundred years.

Advocacy within nursing has had such great role models as Florence Nightingale, the nurse who revolutionized the delivery of health care services to soldiers during the Crimean War and who defined and founded nursing as it is known today, and Margaret Sanger, the internationally known founder of the birth control movement in the United States. More recently, gerontological nurses have claimed that the unique specialty of gerontological nursing is generalization and not specialization. All of these point to nursing's role in coordinating services within institutional settings, within community settings, and among settings during periods of transition, as from the hospital to the home.

Mediation is also a nursing role that has both micro and macro elements. For instance, at the micro level, the nurse interprets an elder's behavior to a critical staff member and negotiates a resolution of the conflicts between the elder and the staff member, or the nurse acts to resolve conflicts between an individual elder and an individual family member. At the macro level, the nurse can interpret the needs of specific groups of elders to bureaucrats in order to negotiate rules and regulations that meet the needs of both the legal system and the group of elders.

With all of these concepts and role responsibilities in mind, it is apparent that nursing has a role in shaping the processes of the care of elderly clients in the community and in institutions. Two special groups that nursing is uniquely qualified to care for deserve special attention: those who are dying and those who have dementing disorders. Two commonalities unite these groups. Both require intensive, virtually continuous care, and both have exhausted their options for cure and must rely almost exclusively on nursing management to meet their needs for comfort, safety, and quality of life.

The role of nursing in the hospice movement is well established, but hospice care is broadly defined by the terminal nature of a specific disease and how close the client is to dying, rather than by age. Integrating traditional hospice concepts with gerontological nursing concepts is an important way that nursing can contribute generally to care of the elderly.

The care of those with dementing illnesses, such as Alzheimer's disease, is often relegated to nurse extenders, as if there were no professional nursing role with these clients. However, a series of nursing studies suggest that, even though dementing disorders are characterized by progressive cognitive decline, the decline in functional status can be slowed through deliberative nursing intervention. The role of nursing in shaping the care process for this special population is unquestionable.

The Nursing Role in Determining Structure

The nursing role in the structure domain of health care for the elderly is not universally recognized for at least two reasons.

First, in the past fifty years, nurses have become viewed as actors within the health care system, particularly in their role as employees, rather than as determinants of the system. Before this time, it was not uncommon for nurses to hold positions as hospital administrators. The majority of nurses were independent contractors who were responsible to their clients for the quality of their care rather than to bureaucratic structures. Now, however, the most common nursing roles, the ones that the public and the paranursing professionals see enacted, involve working within the present system as agents of the prevailing power structure. In addition, the intimate primary relationship that developed in the past between a nurse and a patient has been replaced by relationships between patients and multiple, often unidentifiable, strangers who perform highly intimate tasks.

Second, as technological advances have reduced death rates from acute illnesses, the importance of nursing care as a primary therapy for avoiding death has been diminished. Before the advent of antibiotics, for example, the most effective, and basically the only, therapies for preventing death from infectious disease were those that were prescribed and administered by nurses. Because technological development is now seen as outside the realm of nursing, and because nursing care is viewed as incidental to recovery, the role of nurses in determining the structure in which highly technological care is provided has come to be viewed as irrelevant.

Although, operationally, the role of nursing in determining the structure of the health care designed to meet the needs of the elderly is negligible, conceptually, there are many reasons supporting the importance of the nursing role.

First, the current service-delivery structure is based on the assumption that the health care needs of the elderly are driven by acute, short-term illnesses that are best treated in hospitals and most adequately described by medical diagnoses. The fact is that chronic, long-term illnesses mostly determine the health care needs of the elderly. These illnesses are best characterized by their effects on self-care activities and emotional states; the most appropriate treatment setting is only occasionally the acute-care hospital. Regardless of the diagnosis involved, however, the need for some level of nursing care is the common denominator that underlies the health care needs of the elderly. Consequently, nursing has an important role in determining the nature of health care structures so that the problems of daily living experienced by the elderly are accorded as much emphasis as other facets of their care.

Second, although the current service-delivery structure assumed that the health needs of the elderly follow the same natural history or trajectory as those of younger populations, they are cyclical instead and more prolonged than those in younger groups. Rehabilitation, for example, is possible following acute illness, but the rehabilitation outcomes are different for younger and elderly groups, and the time required for rehabilitation is longer for the elderly.

For many elderly clients, health problems are never absent regardless of the medical treatment; they only go through cycles of "better" or "worse." For example, an elder with chronic lung disease is never free of the disease and never really well. During the "better" phase of the cycle she or he may be able to perform daily living tasks such as bathing and dressing with relative ease and, with support, successfully manage at home. Because the line between "better" and "worse" is so fragile, however, the "worse" phase of the cycle can be triggered by simple things such as stress or fatigue, both of which are potentially avoidable to some degree. A cascade of physiological events may occur that leads to repeated hospitalizations that might have been prevented given a carefully planned stress-management–energy-conservation program. Prolonged or frequent periods of "worse" can result in long-term institutionalization as informal supports, such as family, become exhausted by the complexity of the care.

Central to meeting the health care needs of the elderly, then, are critical issues such as continuity of care among treatment settings, monitoring and supporting the client and the family to suppress the triggers that worsen health problems, and adapting treatment environments to maximize function. Prevention of iatrogenic illnesses (those brought on by the treatment itself) and premature functional decline is also crucial. Nursing roles such as those of the nurse case manager, the home health nurse, the community health nurse, the gerontological clinical specialist, and the geriatric nurse practitioner are designed to address these critical issues. Nursing, therefore, can shape the service delivery structure to accommodate those roles that are likely to meet the special health-care needs of the elderly within and between settings and can at the same time, reduce the cost of care by helping the elder to avoid costly high-tech interventions.

A third reason for the importance of the nursing role in determining structure is simply that a majority of the health care needs of the elderly are nursing-care needs. Because these needs are related to problems of everyday living (e.g., bathing, eating, ambulating, and self-medicating), it is assumed that few specialized skills are required by those who provide the nursing care. As a consequence, the majority of the individuals who provide nursing care to the elderly are not professional nurses. Rather, they are usually nursing assistants or untrained family members.

The degree to which the care of nonnurses actually meets the needs of the elderly for nursing care varies widely. Interestingly, when the amount of time that the professional nurse spends providing direct services to the elderly is increased, there is a significant improvement in care outcomes. For example, the Robert Wood Johnson Teaching Nursing Home Project recently demonstrated that, in the institutional setting, when geriatric nurse practitioner time was provided, there was a decrease in hospitalizations as well as other improvements in selected outcomes, such as a decreased use of urinary catheters, decreased incontinence, a decreased use of both physical and chemical restraints, a reduced prevalence of infection and falls, and a decline in pressure sores.

In short, nursing has an important role in determining the allocation of the human resources required for meeting the health care needs of the elderly. In addition, nursing has a role in the policy decisions regarding staffing ratios and case mix, in the recruitment and retention of nurse extenders, and in the education of those who are actually meeting the nursing-care needs of the elderly, including family caregivers.

The Nursing Role in Defining Outcomes

The notion of professional accountability for the outcomes of care is a fairly new one. Until recently, morbidity and mortality statistics (the incidence of disease and death) have served as the primary means of measuring outcomes. The links between professionally provided care and morbidity and mortality have been very loose because of the number of uncontrollable factors involved, such as genetic predisposition and lack of knowledge about prevention.

The recent interest in defining outcome measures and linking these directly to professionally provided care has arisen for several reasons. First, with technological advancement, it is within the realm of possibility, for the first time, to actually implement interventions aimed at preventing morbidity and mortality and to measure the outcomes. Second, social forces have raised the notion that our health-care system should provide "health for all." In addition, current modes of communication allow observers to track the degree to which "health for all" actually exists. Third, political and economic forces have created a climate in which the federal government is becoming less willing to accept the financial responsibility for expensive, unsuccessful treatment. Now, the health care community is faced with the task of defining the outcomes for which it is truly possible to be held accountable. This task is tremendously challenging and has yet to be accomplished.

The notion of outcomes is extremely tricky with regard to care of the elderly. The traditional outcome measures of morbidity and mortality are very problematic for this group. No amount of intervention is going to eliminate death, although, even when individuals are in their nineties, the concept of preventable or premature death is still relevant. On one level, the concept of illness prevention may seem meaningless because, even if the individual sustains health throughout his or her lifetime, the inevitable outcome of life (which is death) always has some illness-based cause, except in the case of accident. The other side of the coin is that, until the ultimate outcome, illness prevention can decrease the incidence of acute illness in the elderly and can result in increased well-being and an improved quality of life despite a continuing chronic illness.

Another factor complicating the notion of outcomes of care in the elderly is the cost of health care and the acceptability of the measures available to prevent mortality at the end of life. For example, although a heart transplant may temporarily prevent the death of a ninety-five-year-old, the cost of the treatment measured against the certainty and stability of the outcome makes it difficult to justify the use of minimally prolonged life as an appropriate outcome. In addition, many elders would not view minimally prolonged life as an appropriate outcome measure given the pain involved.

Nursing has several very special contributions to make in defining the outcomes of health care for the elderly. Quality of life, for example, is an outcome measure that has become generally accepted as appropriate for the elderly. Quality of life is directly associated with the problems of everyday existence. Because nursing is particularly involved in this dimension of care, it can contribute knowledge of the special daily-living problems of the elderly to the identification of the parameters of quality of life. In a recent study, a number of elders, family members, and case managers were interviewed in an effort to identify the outcomes of nurse case management. Many of the elders interviewed identified their abilities to help others and to make meaningful contributions to family and society (both of which are developmental tasks associated with aging) as outcomes that had resulted from a nurse's assisting them to regain their functional abilities. Both abilities were viewed by the elders as essential to maintaining the quality of their lives. Because of nursing's role in providing intimate and sustained care to elders and their families, nurses have a special vantage point from which to witness how care changes quality of life. As a consequence, many of the as-yet-unidentified dimensions of quality of life can be identified and defined by nursing.

Costs, also, have been used as outcome measures of the quality of care. The focus on costs has been the impetus for the emphasis on community-based care for even acutely ill elders. Because of nursing's role in providing home care, it has a unique perspective on the human costs with regard to dimensions such as disintegrating family systems, which are not often considered in traditional cost analyses.

Based on these examples, it is clear that nursing has important contributions to make in the area of outcome definition. It is absolutely imperative that nursing's role be used as health-care-policy organizations search for appropriate outcomes and as individual agencies develop systems of evaluating the care being provided.

Conclusion

Nursing has a role in direct service delivery to the elderly and in the shaping of the health care system that will provide direct services to the elderly in the future. The domains, or facets, of nursing's role include process, structure, and outcome.

One additional facet has yet to be discussed. The role of nursing in developing the knowledge base underlying health care delivery to the elderly is increasingly apparent. Currently, the knowledge base underlying geriatric and gerontological practice is advanced in some areas and primitive in others. We have fairly good descriptions of the nature of the problems commonly encountered by the elderly and the scope of these problems. Our data are clear about the demographic trends that are driving health-care-delivery systems and about the types of problems that are likely to occur in the future. In addition, we have a fair amount of knowledge about the treatment of various illnesses, although there is a great deal still to be learned in many areas (e.g., dementing disorders and chronic cardiovascular diseases). On the whole, however, we have very little information about the nature of the aging experience from the perspective of the individual client and family. Few research data are available on the additive effects of facing multiple chronic health problems over time.

The research to date has failed to take into account an integrated view of the health problems of the elderly. The problems of everyday life and the ways of reducing those problems are poorly researched, as are the ways of promoting personal integrity and growth among progressively frailer patients and families.

Nursing has special knowledge in all of these areas. Although the research-based knowledge underlying nursing practice is still developing, nurse-researchers have an important role in describing, testing, and refining the nonmedical interventions that nurses regularly use and the various models that currently drive nursing practice. They also have the collaborative role in research of testing the applicability and efficacy of service delivery models.

In sum, nursing has many important roles in relation to shaping the processes, structures, and outcomes of the care of the elderly. In addition, nursing has a role in systematically developing and testing, through research, the knowledge base needed to improve health care for the elderly in the future.

8

Changing Health Needs and Medical Education for the Future

THOMAS LANGFITT, M.D.

> My remarks in this chapter center on the following theme: The health care needs of the American people are changing and will continue to change in the years ahead, but the philosophy that is the educational foundation for the health professions, especially the profession of medicine, and the ways in which health professionals are educated and trained are out of step with the changing health needs of the people.

First, in what ways are health needs changing? We see them every day in our personal lives and in our practices.

The population is aging. In 1900, 30 percent of the people who were born in 1830 were still alive at age seventy. But in 1980, 80 percent of the people born in 1910 were still alive at age seventy. To my mind, this is a more compelling way to demonstrate how much longer people are living than the usual life-expectancy figures.

Improvements in infant mortality have much to do with improvements in total mortality, as we all know. Infant mortality rates are now just above 10 deaths per 1,000 live births. Dramatic as that improvement is, we need to remember that this figure ranks the United States about twentieth among the nations of the world; infant mortality rates in North Philadelphia and in counties of the Mississippi Delta, for example, are 25 to 30 per 1,000 live births.

As people are living longer, what do they look like as they age? They are certainly functioning at a lower capacity than they were when they were younger. Indeed, when I see how steep the lines are in Figure 1, I find it remarkable that I am doing as well as I am.

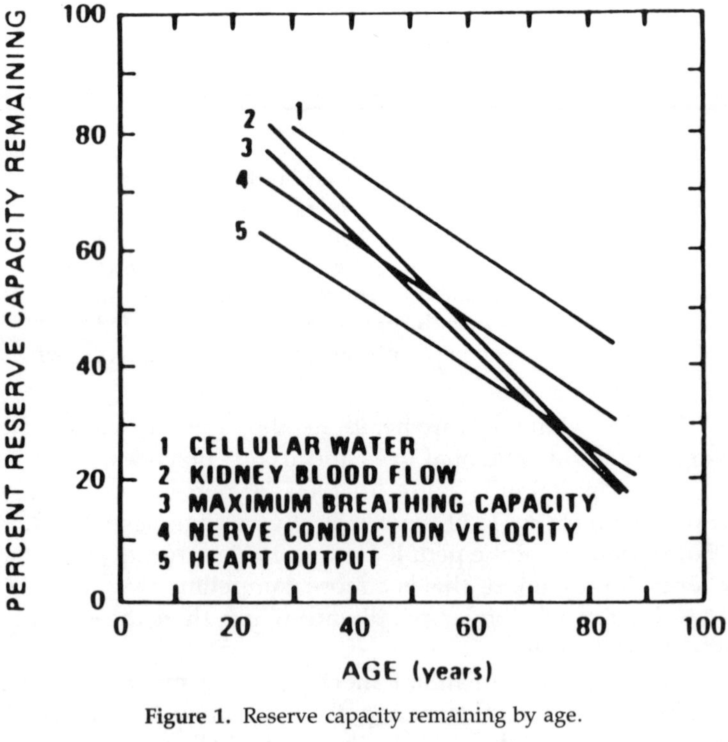

Figure 1. Reserve capacity remaining by age.

Table 1. Morbidity Associated with Senescence: Risk Factors in Parentheses

Cataracts and corneal opacification[a]
Hearing loss[a]
Osteoporosis[b] (inactivity, diet)
Falls and fractures[b] (multiple)
Memory loss[b] (disuse, drugs)
Senile dementia
Incontinence
Constipation[a] (inactivity, diet)
Iatrogenic problems[b] (polypharmacy)
Dependence[b] (multiple)

[a]Effective treatment often possible.
[b]Importantly preventable with present knowledge.

Table 1 shows the morbidity, types of diseases, associated with the process of growing older, senescence, and progressive frailty.

What challenges do we face in managing a larger and larger population with these sorts of problems? The role of specific medical and surgical interventions will continue to be very large. These interventions include surgery for cataracts and a benign enlarged prostate; pharmaceuticals for hypertension, arrhythmias, and cardiac failure; joint replacements; the early diagnosis and treatment of cancer; and many more.

But as I discuss in more detail below, we will be called on more and more to demonstrate the efficacy of these interventions measured by clinical outcomes. How many elderly patients with cataracts are operated on too early? How many times must a man get up at night to go to the bathroom before he should take the small risk of impotence and incontinence that may follow a resection of the prostate? And what about the efficacy of risky and very expensive operations, such as coronary bypass surgery or the surgical removal of an arteriosclerotic plaque of the carotid artery.

Table 2 illustrates the kind of changes in mind set and direction that I believe the members of the health care system will

Table 2. Necessary Changes

Process to outcome
Palliation to prevention
Physical sciences to behavioral sciences
Hospital to home
Authority to advocate

need to adopt in order to meet the changing health-care needs of the people, and particularly the elderly.

A Change in Direction for Medical Education

The second part of my theme declares that education and training for the health professions lag behind this changing landscape of health-care needs. This is most true of medicine and much less true of nursing and dentistry, in my opinion. Allied health is a mixed bag because it contains so many different disciplines. Pharmacy seems to be divided by its educational goals, or at least the education required to achieve those goals. I gather that public health is in the process of casting some fresh light on its mission. Although veterinary medicine does not contribute directly to human health care, of all the professions I believe its leaders have been most willing to work together to define what the needs of veterinary medicine are and how to serve those needs.

I will concentrate now on medicine, because physicians continue to drive the health care system, and in my opinion, the education and training of physicians are of greatest concern within the present context.

How is medicine taught today? Curricula vary from school to school, and some curricula are changing, rather dramatically toward the objectives I have described. But for the most part, curricula consist of two years of basic biomedical sciences, often with clinical diagnosis and some exposure to patients in the second year, and the third and fourth years are divided into a large number of four- to eight-week required and elective rotations.

The students spend most of their time on the hospital floors and some of their time in the outpatient department. Because they are taught almost entirely by specialists and because of the nature of the hospital population today, the orientation is toward organ-based, episodic, crisis-oriented medicine. The students usually do not follow up their patients for any length of time. Therefore, they do not understand the principles and practice of continuity of care that are at the heart of nearly all medical practice.

With this exposure to progressively more specialization in medical school, most students then enter postgraduate specialty training, where they get more of the same. Most of the residents spend most of their time on the hospital floors; often, they do not have any ongoing responsibility for the patients they have managed in the hospital, and altogether, they are not trained to understand and manage an office practice, which is where most of them will spend most of their professional lives.

What I have just described is mainly process. What about the content of education and training for medicine? Table 3 gives an incomplete list of subjects that, to my mind, are as important for physicians to know as is much of the basic and clinical science to which they are exposed during the course of their education and training. Many of these subjects can be taught just as well, or better, in premedical education.

To add even more controversy to my comments, I would make room for some of these subjects by further integration and shortening of the curriculum in the basic biomedical sciences, by eliminating some specialty rotations and by reducing the total number of elective courses through a limitation on specialty electives.

Table 3. Subjects for the New Curriculum

Social sciences	Clinical decision making
Behavioral sciences	Community-based care
Epidemiology	Outcome management
Ethics	History of health care

The purpose of curricular changes such as these would be to place greater emphasis on an understanding of the needs of the whole patient and to teach and train physicians in settings comparable to the settings in which they will practice. I am not making a judgment, at least not now, about how many physicians we need in the specialties compared to the number we need in primary care, the initial entry into the health care system. But I am expressing the belief that an understanding of the issues I have presented thus far is as important for the specialists as it is for the generalists.

Experiment in New Mexico

Ten years ago, the medical school of the University of New Mexico began an experiment that was designed to encourage students to enter community practice. I believe that experiment is relevant to our discussion.

New Mexico is a thinly populated, largely rural state that has had limited health care available outside the three population centers in the state. In 1972, New Mexico ranked forty-ninth among the fifty states in the number of primary-care physicians per 1,000 population. The University of New Mexico School of Medicine is the only medical school in the state, and four-fifths of each graduating class were leaving the state to practice elsewhere. The experiment included three innovations:

- Clinical problem-based learning instead of lecture-based learning
- Student-centered instead of faculty-centered learning
- Community-oriented learning, introduced to complement hospital-oriented learning

The new curriculum began in 1979 with twenty students, out of a total of about one hundred students per class. The most radical change was initiated in the first year of the curriculum.

The initial six-month, on-campus phase of the program is

organized around an integration of basic and clinical science themes. That is, the students do not start with traditional basic science courses consisting of lectures, seminars, and laboratories. Instead, from the beginning, they learn their basic sciences in conjunction with patients who have specific diseases and disorders. For example, in the first week, the students might see a jaundiced patient and then would study the basic sciences by exploring a range of issues associated with liver disease: bilirubin metabolism in biochemistry; histology, or tissue structure and organization, of the liver in anatomy; the circulation of the liver in physiology; viral infections in microbiology; sexual practices in behavioral science; and populations at risk for hepatitis in epidemiology.

During the second half of the first year, the students are placed in a primary-care clinic. Community health experience is intended to balance the tertiary care, hospital-based experiences that will come later in their education. They are assigned to rural areas and work under carefully selected internists, pediatricians, and family physicians. Their goals are to apply the self-directed, problem-based learning skills that they began to acquire the first half of the year to real-life settings in the company of community-physician role models.

The second year, the third year, and half of the fourth year follow the conventional medical school curriculum. Learning is organ-based, and most of the students' time is spent on the hospital floors. However, during the fourth year, the students return to a rural community to apply their newly learned clinical skills with a broader perspective in an extended preceptorship. In effect, there is a fundamental change in about one-fourth of the medical school curriculum.

What differences can be measured between the students in the primary-care curriculum and their classmates who have paralleled them through four years of medical school in the conventional curriculum?

On Part I of the National Board, the primary-care students scored lower, with a mean score of about 425 compared to just over 500 for those on the conventional track. On Part II of the National Board, however, the students on the community-care track scored higher than the students on the conventional track, with a mean score of 500 compared to 460.

The evaluators of the program also conducted a study of student stress levels by using Kellner's Symptom Questionnaire, which assesses depression, physical symptoms, hostility, and anxiety and yields a total distress score. At the beginning of medical school, there was no difference between the two cohorts. In the second semester, however, the distress score among the students on the conventional track was nearly twice that of those on the community-care track. By graduation, that difference had narrowed, but the distress score was still significantly higher among the conventional-track students.

And finally, what kinds of careers did the students choose? Among all students who entered medical school stating that they wished to practice family medicine, 42 percent on the community-care track did so, compared to 29 percent on the conventional track. Among students who switched their career preference to family medicine from other specialty preferences, 39 percent came from the community-care track and 14 percent from the conventional track. In other words, in this one medical school, the alternative curriculum works—not completely—but substantially.

Several years ago, the Pew Charitable Trusts and the Rockefeller Foundation launched a program, entitled "Health of the Public," that gives support to the University of New Mexico medical school to expand its curriculum throughout the class and, very importantly, into postgraduate medical education. The program also supports five other medical schools in beginning the same general kind of process.

All of us recognize the diversity of American medical schools and the differences between a relatively new medical school that is the major source of physicians for a largely rural state and long-standing, research-oriented urban schools. Nevertheless, one of the boldest curricular reforms in the nation is taking place through the New Pathway Program at the Harvard Medical School, and the Johns Hopkins Medical School is one of the six institutions in the Pew–Rockefeller program.

Clinical Outcome Management

Most of the rest of this chapter discusses clinical outcome management, because I think it is the wave of the future in the practice of medicine and in the other health professions. I believe that the time has come to teach medical students outcome management as part of the curricular reform I have been describing. Indeed, I think it could be a major stimulus to the kind of reform discussed here.

What does the term mean? Paul Ellwood, who coined it, gave the following definition:

> Outcomes management is a technology of patient experience designed to help patients, payers, and providers make rational medical care-related choices based on better insight into the effect of these choices on the patient's life.

Outcome management uses four techniques:

1. It places greater reliance on standards and guidelines that physicians can use in selecting appropriate interventions.
2. It routinely and systematically measures the general functioning and well-being of patients, along with disease-specific clinical outcomes, at appropriate time intervals.
3. An outcome management system pools clinical data on a massive scale.
4. Results are analyzed and disseminated from each segment of the data base and communicated to the appropriate decision makers.

Outcome management takes the concept of the clinical trial of therapeutic efficacy, testing the effectiveness of a drug or a procedure, and puts it into the offices of all physicians so that they are doing clinical trials and observing the results in their practices every day.

The process teaches physicians how to evaluate and record the management of individual patients so that they have ready access to the clinical outcomes of all of their patients in each of the disease categories they diagnose and treat. If they treat patients with diabetes, for example, they use standardized instruments for recording the history, the physical examination, and the diagnostic studies performed; they then record, in a standard format, the treatment of the patient over time and, at intervals, the patient's clinical status. In this way, they are able to assess the clinical outcomes produced by the medical management of their patients, again using standardized formats for recording outcomes. All of this is done on computer terminals, personal computers on the physicians' desks, which are linked to their personal data bases. Physicians no longer write or dictate notes on their patients, and in time, traditional patient files will disappear. All information is in the data base and is immediately accessible to the physicians.

Let us say that, for the next five years, a physician sees 100 new patients with a diagnosis of diabetes. He records information on the patients, and the computer processes the information in formats that permit him to have at his fingertips any analysis he wishes on that population of patients. That information may be how various diabetic syndromes are distributed among the patients, insulin requirements by category of disease, complications of the disease and the treatment of each, and the clinical status of all patients, again recorded in ways that permit the physician to make comparisons across the patient population. He no longer has to guess about results.

Without such a data base, I might discuss a particular diabetic syndrome with a colleague and say that I had seen a half dozen patients with the syndrome; in fact, I might well have seen two dozen. Or I might say I have had a particular complication once or twice in the past ten years when, in fact, I might have had the complication much more frequently, but I do not like complications, so I forget most of them.

The point is that, unless we have the means to analyze our practices, accurately and quantitatively, we do not have a clear idea of what our experiences have been. None of this substitutes for clinical judgment. What it does is honestly record those wise judgments so they are not lost to the practitioner or to posterity.

Once we have in place a system for recording and analyzing

patient information far more accurately than we do today, the next step is clinical outcome management.

How do current practitioners know whether their experiences with diabetes are similar to the experiences of other physicians, and in particular, how do they know whether the outcomes of the treatment of their patients are good, bad, or indifferent compared to those of others? They learn about these things in time-honored ways: from the literature, from local and national meetings, from grand rounds, over coffee, and so on. But they receive that information in a fragmentary way and store it alongside their personal experiences in their memory banks, memory banks that may have some loose wires here and there and are sometimes subject to convenience.

What physicians do in this new mode of practice is compare their experiences from their own data banks with the experiences of colleagues in the same practice in the same hospital and more widely in the same community, and ultimately, they make comparisons with a national data base on diabetes. All of this is done quickly and conveniently, and the information is accurate if the data entered by each practitioner is accurate. So practitioners learn something new every day by comparing their patient management with patient management by countless other physicians. In this way, all of the physicians in the network are learning to manage their patients to better and better outcomes because they are continually sharing their experiences.

What are the risks of a system such as this one? The most obvious risk is that the results obtained by each practitioner are there for everyone to see, at least potentially. Not only might the information be used in legal actions, but if the results are not as good as the results of colleagues down the street, practices may be compromised. Guarding the privacy of the information, therefore, is an essential requirement, one that may be very difficult to meet.

Also, busy practitioners may find the system too cumbersome and time-consuming and may refuse to join. But I have argued that the system would be far simpler and more convenient to use than current practices. Or worse, they may use the system and not do so conscientiously, the result being the garbage-in–garbage-out data syndrome. The system also adds initial expense to the practice, but one can argue that it is only a matter of time before all physicians' offices will be computerized, and a system such as this one could be made also to manage the business affairs of the practice.

As attractive as clinical outcome management may be to many physicians, I am pessimistic about inducing large numbers of physicians now in practice to use it. It is a whole new way of doing things that will take substantial effort, and there is no doubt that it is threatening in some ways.

So although I urge physicians to adopt outcome management in their practices, I believe we should introduce the concept into the medical school curriculum so that all future physicians will learn to practice medicine in these ways. This approach will take longer, but if we really believe in it, I think this is the surer way.

Outcome Management in the Curriculum

I will now describe briefly how outcome management might fit into the medical school curriculum. Students arrive with personal computers compatible with the outcome management system in the medical center. During a start-up phase, a system would have been developed and tested in several clinical departments, such as medicine, surgery, and pediatrics. Consequently, physicians in those departments are practicing outcome management when the first cohort of medical students arrive.

In the first year, the students are taught the concepts of outcome management. They learn how to enter clinical information into the data base, how to assess health status, and how to manage information on populations of patients, including appropriate statistics and other subject matter that will prepare them for their first exposure to patients. The course extends throughout the first year and parallels the basic science courses in schools with conventional curricula.

In the second year, the students begin to see patients and to learn clinical diagnosis in an outcome format. From the beginning, they learn how to make clinical observations in standardized formats—in principle, not much different from the ways students now learn to take a history and do a physical examination—and they begin to learn how to compare groups of patients with the same disorder.

In the third year, they begin to develop their own practices. Very importantly, they cannot learn to practice outcome management if they see the patients only during hospital admission or only hit-or-miss in the outpatient department. Continuity of care is critical for the outcome-management learning process, and that is the way most physicians practice in the real world, yet it is also one of the greatest shortcomings of both undergraduate and graduate medical education today. So outcome management forces continuity of care by its insistence on the on-going care of substantial numbers of patients throughout the last two years of medical school.

After graduation from medical school, the students continue the same practices in postgraduate training. When they have completed training, they practice outcome management because that is the only way they know how to practice.

If all this should come to pass what would have been accomplished?

First, physicians would better understand their long-term responsibilities to their patients.

Second, physicians would better understand the composition of their practices and the results of the diagnostic and treatment modalities, or methods, they use.

Third, they would be in a position to continually improve the management of their patients by continually comparing their experiences with those of their colleagues.

Fourth, the system provides an intellectual underpinning to the practice of medicine that does not exist today. Every practitioner will become a clinical investigator.

Fifth, the public benefits because medicine is practiced more intelligently, with greater benefit and less risk to the patients.

Sixth, money is saved because physicians practicing the

same specialty are able to identify the most effective ways of managing patients. They can also identify procedures to be abandoned because they have been demonstrated to be ineffectual.

Commission on the Future of the Health Professions

I close with a description of the Commission on the Future of the Health Professions that is being established by the Pew Trusts to address the issues we have been discussing here. The premise on which the commission is based is that the health care system is in deep distress. In a recent public survey 89 percent of American respondents stated that the health care system needed fundamental reform. In contrast, 63 percent of British respondents and only 43 percent of Canadians stated that their systems needed fundamental reform. It is interesting that the expenditures for health care in the United States are 12 percent of the gross national product, compared to 8 percent in Canada and 6 percent in Great Britain.

So there seems to be a strong consensus that some kind of fundamental change must take place within our system. Tinkering around the edges will no longer work. The key issues now are costs and access to the system. Currently, indemnity premiums paid by companies for their employees are increasing by 20 to 35 percent per year and are creating more of an outcry from the corporate community than we have heard for a long time. Many small companies are being priced out of the market, and the underwriting practices used by some insurance companies are excluding many self-employed people who can still afford insurance.

All of this is compounding the problem of access to the system. We hear repeatedly about the thirty to forty million poor, including working poor, Americans who do not have health insurance. The Pepper Commission, established to address the problems of health care, recently issued its report amid great expectations. It calculated that coverage for the uninsured poor would cost $85 billion, on top of the current health-care budget, which is approaching $700 billion, but it had no constructive suggestions about where to find the money.

Those who practice medicine know what is happening on the expense side of the ledger. The federal government and other payers are attempting to control hospital charges, physicians' fees, and the use of the health care system in any way they can. More and more, this attempt at control takes the decision-making process about the patient away from physicians and increases their practice expenses with a myriad of reporting requirements. This combination of pressures has produced more anger, anxiety, and dissatisfaction than we have ever seen within the medical profession. Applications to medical schools are down, and in a recent survey of physicians conducted by the American Medical Association, only 24 percent said they definitely would enter medicine today if they had it all to do over again.

The recommendations that I have described are not a fundamental reform of the system; they are a far cry from it. Because costs are the issue, the system is being squeezed by third-party payers without much regard to what will happen within the system. Payers and the public say that they have been frustrated by fifteen years of escalating costs, which have not been contained by prospective payment or competition through managed care. They vent that frustration by attempting to clamp down on the amount of money flowing into the system, whatever the consequences.

What, then, do we mean by fundamental reform? To my mind it must begin with examining the ways in which health care is organized and delivered to the public. In the long run, it must be based on primary-care givers—physicians, nurses, and other health professionals—who are responsible for a defined population of patients and who are advocates for their patients and the gatekeepers for their patients to the rest of the system. We must eliminate the extraordinarily wasteful practice of patients' passing from specialist to specialist, without guidance, and consuming more and more resources with unnecessary and repetitious diagnostic and therapeutic procedures. And that is only one example of the waste that occurs in what is a health care nonsystem.

Our national Commission on the Education for the Health Professions will begin its deliberations by asking the following questions of itself:

1. Are there ways in which health care can be provided to all Americans at affordable prices within the current system? If they find the answer to the question, we can disband the commission and enshrine all members in the pantheon of great American heroes.
2. What would a system look like that would achieve those objectives of cost containment and access and would also be acceptable to both health care providers and the public? I think you would agree that that system would require a considerable change in mind-set on the part of both physicians and patients.

Recall my opening remarks: "The philosophy that is the educational foundation for the health professions, especially the profession of medicine, and the ways in which health professionals are educated and trained are out of step with the changing health needs of the people."

That is a premise on my part, and the issue will be put to the commission in the form of the following questions:

- Once we have defined the health needs of the population, ranging from primary care through the most complex tertiary care for all ages and for all groups at risk, is the education and training of health professionals appropriate to serve those needs?
- If there is a disparity between education and training and need, what can be done about it?
- Specifically, can we design a system that would reform education and training for all of the health professions, where reform is needed, so that, over time, physicians and other health professionals entering the system will be meeting the health needs of the people better than current practitioners are able to do?

- And finally, can we illustrate how those changes will contribute to a system that will provide access to health care for all people at affordable prices?

Given the magnitude of that challenge, I am surprised that so many distinguished Americans have agreed to serve on the commission.

II

SOCIAL AND PSYCHOLOGICAL ISSUES

9

Families of the Aged

An Overview of Family Caregiving

BARBARA SILVERSTONE, D.S.W.

As recently as two decades ago, the topic of family caregiving for an aging relative received little attention in either professional or lay circles. Today, when such caregiving is a reality for so many families, the topic has become commonplace in both discussion and research. It is regarded, says social worker Elaine Brody, as a "normative family stress,"[1] an everyday part of life for many families. In this chapter I summarize the accumulated knowledge about family caregiving for the elderly and discuss its implications for policy and practice, emphasizing the pivotal role played by social workers in each of these areas.

The Modified Extended Family

Most older persons in our society are integrated into multigenerational family structures, not separated by isolated nuclear family units as many had once thought. In this modified extended family, although most older persons tend to live in separate households from the younger generations, they are clearly full-fledged members within the family structure.

Despite dramatic shifts in the family structure since the turn of the century, the model of the modified family still holds true. Families now encompass more generations because of the growing number of persons surviving into old age, but they have fewer members within each generation because of a decreasing fertility rate.

To illustrate, 10 percent of those now over the age of sixty-five have living children also over the age of sixty-five. Of the elderly, 70 percent are grandparents, and 40 percent are great-grandparents. At the other end of the spectrum, in 1970 the American family had an average of 2.6 children, compared to 4.5 in 1910.

Elders are generally satisfied with their relationships with family and friends, but for the most part, they tend to live apart as married couples or alone, although close to their children. For the young-old (usually sixty-five to seventy-five), the most typical living arrangement is with a spouse. Only one in six of the elderly, aged sixty-five and over shares a dwelling with an adult child. Although the majority of elders do not *choose* to live with their children, the likelihood that they will increases for both men and women in the very late years, paralleling the increase in institutionalization. Of very old men (eighty-five and older), 14 percent live with a child, as do 26 percent of very old women.

The elderly do not appear to be socially isolated even though most families live in separate generational households. Most elderly parents see their children often or maintain contact by telephone or mail. Of those with children, 80 percent report seeing them at lest once a week, and 70 percent live within a thirty-minute drive of a child. This intensity of contacts between adult children and their aging parents has been characterized as "intimacy at a distance." When friends and neighbors are added to the social network of the elderly, the likelihood of isolation becomes even more remote.

Multigenerations: Impact on the Family

What has been the impact on the family of these widespread, relatively intense intergenerational relationships? An increasing number of gerontologists view the overall impact as positive, noting more complexity in family networks, including "relationships of unprecedented duration, decades of shared experience, and the opportunity to forge new roles."[2]

The economic improvements experienced by older persons in recent decades have contributed heavily to this positive impact. Increased government and retirement pensions and health care provisions have dramatically reduced the financial burden of elderly parents on adult children. Now only 9 percent of the elderly receive regular financial help from their children and only 3 to 4 percent occasional help. This dramatic decrease in financial dependency between the generations, in the opinion of some experts, accounts for the abundance of nonfinancial social exchanges. It appears that the diminished strain eases the relationship and makes other interactions more desirable.

In the majority of extended families, elders and their adult children participate in a mutual exchange of goods and services, although the participation of elders tends to decrease as they become more frail or impaired. These private transfers are receiving increased attention in the gerontological community as the controversy over generational inequity in government funding swells. In a national survey some time ago, 90 percent of a sample of Americans over the age of sixty-five reported helping younger family members with child care, other services, and gifts of money. There were even people seventy-five and over continuing to provide support to younger generations. On the other hand, older persons with families benefit by the extensive care and support they can usually count on when and if frailty and impairment strike. The extent of family care for the elderly has been well documented. Families provide 80 percent of all home health care for older people.

Quality of Intergenerational Relations

Although the objective circumstances (i.e., living arrangements, number of contacts, and kinds of exchanges) in the relationships between adult children and their aging parents can be described, the quality of and satisfaction in those relationships are harder to measure. The limited knowledge accumulated to date suggests that affection and trust between the generations generally appears to be strong, and adult children are often viewed as confidants by their elderly parents.

Bengston and Kuypers found that adult children and aging parents have differing perspectives and expectations of their relationship. The elderly report higher levels of affection in their relationships than their children do, and they minimize, in contrast to their children, the exchange of services. A research study in the Netherlands corroborated the findings of Bengston and Kuypers but found that, although the generations seemed to disagree much of the time, most parents and children did not perceive these differences as applying to their own relationships. Instead, both groups apparently work hard at minimizing their differences in order to maintain a sense of solidarity, cohesiveness, and continuity.

These factors seem to dominate most relationships between older parents and their adult children. They shape family perceptions and affect family roles, as evidenced in the mediating role that adult children assume on behalf of aging parents. Adult children often serve as go-betweens with physicians and other professionals and are generally helpful in coping with the crises of old age.

The once-popular notion of role reversal between the generations was first criticized by social work clinician Sonja Rhodes, who suggested instead that the concepts of mutual aid and reciprocity more nearly describe the relationship. Increasing attention is being given by family therapists to the multiple effects of intergenerational issues on family dynamics.

The Caregiving Situation

Social work researcher Amy Horowitz differentiates the caregiving relationship from other family exchanges, noting that it is "defined by the existence of some degree of physical, mental, emotional, or economic impairment on the part of the older person which limits independence and necessitates ongoing assistance."[3] The variability in caregiving behavior among families, although an important subject of ongoing and future research, is not seen as the decisive factor in determining if care will be provided or not. Rather, the needs of the elder are the determining factor in both whether and how much care will be provided.

The primary caregiver is generally the spouse, if there is one available, and a child, if there is not. In the absence of both spouse and children, other relatives take on some responsibility. Spouses give the most comprehensive care and also report the highest levels of stress. Although adult children also tend to be extensively involved in and affected by caregiving, their involvement is less intense, although a strong bond appears to exist in most caregiving relationships.

Females predominate over males as primary caregivers. Because men tend to marry younger women and women outlive men, the usual caregiver for an older man is his wife and for an older woman is her daughter, who faces competing responsibilities from family and/or employment. Close proximity seems to determine which adult child in a family will be the one to care for an aging parent.

Caregiving activities vary widely among families and range from occasional errands to round-the-clock care for the bedridden; the time spent ranges from an average of three hours a week to well over forty. Families do not specialize or concentrate help in any one or two areas but increase services to meet needs as they arise. Much of this variation, as noted previously, appears to be a function of the older person's impairment. Emotional support is the most universal caregiving task engaged in by almost every caregiver. It includes maintaining social interaction and "cheering up" the depressed older person.

The economic costs of caregiving to the family, at least in the United States, cannot be minimized. Though there is generally an equal exchange of goods and services between the generations, when older people become frail and impaired caregiving *per se* entails great economic cost to the family. A comprehensive study of the cost comparison of home care found that family and friends were absorbing the largest portion of the cost of long-term care, compared to the expenditure of public dollars. As stated previously, families provide 80 percent of all home health care for older people, and conversely, 80 percent of all older people with home-health-care needs depend primarily on their family.

The critical importance of family care is underscored by the fact that, for each older resident, in a nursing home, there are two in the community with similar disabilities being cared for by family. Widows, those living alone, and those without children are the most likely to enter nursing homes. Older people with family support tend to enter nursing homes at much higher levels of impairment than those who enter without family support because their families tend to care for them as long as possible. Exhaustion of family resources, excessive burden, and change in family circumstances, more often than change in the older person's health status, are the primary causes of nursing-home placement. Some families reach a crisis when they can no longer provide the care needed by an older relative. This fact, in combination with increasingly outspoken coalitions of family caregivers, has focused a great deal of attention on the negative effects of caregiving on the health and general well-being of family members.

The Effects of Caregiving on the Caregiver

In studies of families currently providing care to an elder, both positive and negative effects are noted. Satisfaction is reported by many caregivers, even in situations where considerable burden is experienced. This finding is not surprising if the broader context of reciprocal, or mutual, family relationships is taken into account. The positive effect of caregiving also serves to discount popular notions that caregiving on the part of adult children is motivated simply by guilt or a sense of duty.

There are also negative effects on the physical and emotional health of family caregivers, such as increased levels of depression and anxiety as well as lower morale. In many adult-child–aging-parent relationships, emotional strain appears to be the greatest burden experienced and is more pervasive and difficult for the caregiver to deal with than with the physical aspects of care.

On a clinical level, there is repeated documentation of the intense emotions stirred by the increased dependency and worsened condition of an aging parent. Margaret Blenkner, a leading social-work researcher, was the first to describe the filial crisis faced by the adult child in relation to the aging parent. The family caregiver most stressed is the female spouse and, next, the adult daughter.

Caregiving for a mentally impaired elder appears to generate the most stress, at times to the extent that physical and mental health are threatened. In a study of London families of elderly persons who resided in hospital geriatric units, those "intolerable" problems that prevented the families from accepting the older persons back into their homes included the disruptive behavior patterns of the elder, the general immobility of the aged person, personal problems such as anxiety or depression generated by the caregiving role, restrictions on social activities, and a change in environmental conditions because of the presence and needs of the elder.

Second only to the emotional strains, and often associated with them, are the restrictions on time and freedom necessitated by caregiving responsibilities and activities. Relatively lower stress is associated with financial concerns, although caregiving may involve financial contributions and may strain the economic resources of the family. Many caregivers give up employment or reduce their work schedule to carry out caregiving tasks.

Yet, the ability of families to cope in spite of burdens and stresses is striking. In the London study, 617 families caring for impaired elders in residence, usually over extended periods of time, seemed to be coping with the responsibilities. Although almost 80 percent of the caregivers reported one or more caregiving tasks as difficult, tiring, or emotionally upsetting, the results indicated that the caregivers, on the whole, were not in *serious* psychological distress. To date, there does not seem to be a widespread or significant reduction in parent care by working women. On the contrary, caregivers may leave employment or reduce their work hours to care for an aging parent. Further, race, ethnicity, and socioeconomic status do not appear to be important variables in explaining differences in caregiver behavior.

Although the severity of the older person's impairment is a key factor in the caregiver's perception of burden, there is not a direct correlation between the two. The degree of involvement and certain characteristics of the caregiver also have an influence. Help, visits, and alternate forms of secondary support from kin are also mitigating factors in the caregiving burden.

The actual, or objective, burdens of caregiving must be differentiated from the perceived, or subjective, burdens, those relating to the caregiver's attitude toward or emotional response to the caregiving experience. The means used to ameliorate the objective burden may not be the same as those needed to relieve the subjective burden, an important consideration in evaluations of intervention strategies.

Quality of Care and Quality of Life

Little is known about the quality of care provided by families and friends to impaired frail elders, and far less is known about the quality of life imposed by the caregiving situation. Although research shows that elders prefer the help of family, questions remain concerning the degree of skill with which families care for the moderately-to-severely impaired elder and the extent of family abuse.

In one of the few in-depth studies to examine these caregiving issues, family members who lived with and cared for their elders reported difficulty in caring for mentally impaired elders, particularly those exhibiting negative behavior. Incontinence and heavy lifting were also problems for the families. Although 91 percent of the elders who could be interviewed generally reported few complaints and stated that they preferred to continue their present arrangement, 90 percent admitted that they were very dependent on their caregivers, and 55 percent complained that their caregivers did too much for them. In addition, 30 percent agreed that their relationship with their caregivers made them feel useless. This population, like some nursing-home residents, might have been experiencing conditions of "excess disability" or functional loss not justified by their actual physical and mental impairments.

The problem of exploitive and aggressive behavior on the part of caregivers toward helpless, frail elders has long been recognized in nursing homes. The focus has broadened to include families and neighbors of elders in the community, where one study found that 10 percent of the elderly experienced threats or acts of violence from their children, and 18 percent of caregivers experienced violence, usually emotional in nature, by elders. The caregiver "abuser" was likely to be a woman in her late fifties or early sixties who had responsibilities to children and grandchildren and also carried the responsibility of caring for a parent in his or her eighties. Abusive tactics were found to be used as a last resort when other conflict-resolution techniques failed. A recent study of a larger Boston sample found that spouses were most likely to be the family abusers of the elderly.

The Role of the Formal Care System: Policy Implications

Current research shows general agreement about the role and effects of caregiving within the family. There is far less evidence or agreement about the role of the formal care system, which includes the health and social agencies that provide services.

Several sets of issues surround the provision of formal care. Does it substitute for family care? Does formal care actually reduce family burden and stress? The issue of whether formal care is qualitatively better than family care has not been addressed, except by those who stress the advantages of nursing-home care for the severely impaired.

Research in the United States to date has had contradictory findings. Although the available evidence indicates that the provision of formal services does not significantly reduce the previous level of care provided by family caregivers, families have said that the provision of formal services does reduce the emotional and physical burden of care.

This disparity in findings may be due to the minimal amount of formal service available. All aspects of formal care provision must be considered when its impact on family stress is measured, including the quality and goal of formal care, its availability and intensity, the degree of trust placed in it by family members, and the feelings generated by relying on outside help.

Because formal services are far more comprehensive in other industrialized countries, cross-national comparisons may offer the best tool for assessing the impact of formal services on family caregiving.

A longitudinal Canadian study of older persons, extending over four years, showed that the formal support system, over time, contributed to improvement in the relationships between the clients and their informal support network, composed of other than spouses or daughters. This was the case even when the relationships had not been markedly close or positive during the years preceding the current crisis. For clients with spouses and daughters, continuing stable support was provided in addition to formal services.

Two competing perspectives have dominated the discussion of policy pertaining to the formal support of family caregivers. One, embraced by some policymakers in the United States, characterizes the family as an "untapped resource." These persons generally fall into two camps: those who see the family as a partial solution to the problem of rising social and health care costs and those who fear that formal services will undermine the care given by the family.

Social-work policy experts register a strong dissent to this view. Rather, they see the family as being overtaxed and requiring an increase in governmental supports that will supplement and not supplant family care. The resolution of these contrasting views is essential to an effective, coherent policy for family caregivers.

Practice Issues

The considerable research findings on family caregiving to date have striking implications for social work practice. To summarize, families appear to experience a significant degree of emotional burden and stress that is not necessarily relieved by concrete services. Clearly, the mental impairment of an elder takes a toll on the family regardless of the degree of concrete respite services. Furthermore, caregiving interweaves with longstanding family dynamics, giving added force to the emotional strain (the subjective burden) experienced by the caregivers.

The clinical theories developed by social workers and corroborated by these findings stress interventions that are responsive to the whole family and the changing needs of its elderly members. They emphasize the need for clinical sensitivity to the depth and complexity of intergenerational relations. Two such theories are the developmental-systems approach to understanding family dynamics across the life cycle, postulated by Tonti and Silverstone, and the related auxiliary-function approach developed by Silverstone and Burack-Weiss.

The developmental-systems approach views the family as a dynamic whole and encompasses both case management and clinical interventions. It takes into account two sometimes contradictory goals of the family: one related to carrying out concrete and non-concrete tasks on behalf of its members and the other related to maintaining a comfortable level of tension within the family system. This approach may necessitate overlooking or neglecting the needs of an individual family member. For example, a family may decide that they cannot provide the care that an aging parent needs because other members of the family need more attention and care.

Practice interventions involve working with the family to shift or expand family boundaries, redefine tasks, and open up new modes of communication for dealing with intolerable levels of family tension. Family group meetings, which should include the older person if he or she is not too impaired, are a preferred vehicle for family communication and for reviewing problem-solving strategies. Caregiving tasks can also be prioritized and shared, and the need for formal services can be evaluated, with consistent consideration given to maintaining a comfortable level of family tension.

The auxiliary-function model of social work practice is also a systems approach, but it focuses more on the distinctive functions that must be carried out to meet the elderly's increasing needs. The depletions and chronic impairments of advanced age create a set of emotional and practical needs that call for a relationship with a significant other whose role is auxiliary in nature, who lends support for as long as, and only as long as, needed. The tasks associated with this role include emotional support and socialization, as well as helping the frail elder with money management, coordination and supervision of services, and advocacy.

The family usually fills the auxiliary role. When there is no family or when the family, for lack of expertise or resources, cannot totally fill the role, then it is shared with a formal system. The role of the service provider thus becomes twofold: to substitute for the family in filling all or part of the auxiliary role, and/or to work directly with the family to enhance its role.

Although families experiencing a caregiving crisis do seek services, few of these are modeled on a systems approach. Social workers comprise the major source of professional help, but usually in the role of case managers who assist the family in developing and monitoring a plan of care for an elder. The growing numbers of private case managers, most of them social workers, reflect the need of families for professional help in planning and caring for older members. Families living at a distance from the older person are often urgently in need of this help. It is unclear to what extent case managers can or should address the family conflicts and emotional issues that invariably accompany the request for help in planning and finding concrete services.

Other Resources

The above discussion points to the broad opportunities for psychotherapeutic interventions with families that include the old, a relatively new clinical population. Besides specific caregiving issues, many other problems need to be addressed. Marital problems, mental health, financial problems, adjustment to the dilemmas of aging, and intergenerational family situations are common concerns. An aging family structure presents compelling challenges to the helping professions. Yet, as pointed out by social work professor Louis Lowy, psychotherapeutic services are limited, as reflected in the caseloads of mental health clinics, family service agencies, and private practitioners. This dearth of services stems partially from the lack of interest of mental health professionals, including social workers, and also from the older families themselves, which, for financial or attitudinal reasons, do not seek these services. As today's younger families grow older, their greater receptivity to mental health care may result in an increased demand for these services.

Another valuable resource available to the families of older persons are self-help groups, which have proliferated in recent years. Under the auspices of the Alzheimer's Association, a network of self-help groups for families of the victims of Alzheimer's disease has sprung up around the nation and has received widespread support. The emotional support and educational services provided to family members by these and other types of groups is significant, and they, in turn, become effective advocates for better services.

Conclusion

This chapter has documented the solidarity and mutuality that characterize the families of the aged. Although the different generations tend to live apart, social contacts are frequent. Underscored are the contributions made by social work researchers in documenting the importance of family ties not only to the elderly, but also to the social work practitioners and policy experts who address their problems. Frail and impaired older persons, particularly, have benefited from the care provided them by family members, usually wives or daughters; emotional support is considered one of the most universal and important caregiving tasks.

Although satisfaction is experienced by many caregivers, negative effects on physical and mental health cannot be ignored. The emotional stresses associated with caregiving are the most pervasive and difficult to deal with and are especially associated with the care of a mentally impaired elder. Secondary support from kin has been found to be an important factor in alleviating the primary caregiver's burden. Although little is known about the quality of care provided by family and friends to impaired frail elders, older people prefer the help of family. Evidence suggests that some families are overprotective, and other evidence reveals the presence of abuse, usually carried out by spouses, in a small percentage of families.

There is much controversy about the role of the formal care system in relation to family caregiving. The evidence to date suggests that formal services do not ease family burden and stress. Yet, little has been done to measure or evaluate the formal services provided to families and the benefits of respite over and above stress reduction. There is an ongoing policy debate about whether formal services substitute for family care or enhance it, and few research studies in this country have helped to illuminate this controversy. Cross-national studies suggest that formal care of elders supplements, rather than substitutes for, family care.

The implications for social work practice emerging from research findings support long-standing clinical observations. The emotional components of caregiving are embedded in a larger context of the family dynamics that have developed and operated over a long period of time. A family-systems approach has proved useful in concrete planning both with older people and their families and about more complicated emotional issues. Yet, there is still much to explore to further understand the adaptation of older families to the caregiving situation, and to understand the problems both related and unrelated to the caregiving itself.

Social and demographic trends, such as the disproportionate growth in the old-old population, the decreasing nuclear family size, and women's increasing labor force participation, raise serious concerns about the family's caregiving capabilities in the future and the effects on the whole family. Although the capacity of poor families to care for their elderly is apparently extensive, growing poverty among today's young population does not portend well for intergenerational exchanges in the future.

There is little question that families' need for services will grow as more older people survive into very old age and frailty. A variety and flexibility of high-quality services, whether involving respite care, psychotherapy, or self-help groups, are essential to meet those needs.

Notes

1. E. M. Brody, "Aged Parents and Aging Children," in *Aging Parents*, ed. P. K. Ragan. Los Angeles: University of Southern California Press, 1979.
2. G. O. Hagestad, "Able Elderly in the Family Context: Changes, Chances, and Challenges," *The Gerontologist*, 27:4 (August 1987).
3. A. Horowitz, "The Role of Families in Providing Long-Term Care to the Frail and Chronically Ill Elderly Living in the Community" in Final Report submitted to the Health Care Financing Administration, Brookdale Center on Aging at Hunter College, New York, New York, 1982.

Suggested Reading

Nancy L. Mace and Peter V. Rabins, *The 36 Hour Day.* Baltimore: Johns Hopkins University Press, 1981.

Florence D. Shelley, *When Your Parents Grow Old* (2nd ed.). New York: Harper & Row, 1988.

Barbara Silverstone and Helen Kandel Hyman, *You and Your Aging Parent: The Modern Family's Guide to Emotional, Physical, and Financial Problems* (3rd ed.). New York: Pantheon, 1989.

10

Health Benefits of Human–Animal Interaction

LEO K. BUSTAD, D.V.M., PH.D.

Introduction

For thousands of years, people have been closely associated with animals and the environment. Recent clinical observations and research results have lent credibility to the centuries-old belief that a close relationship between people and the natural environment, including animals and plants, is vital to the overall health and well-being of our planet and its inhabitants and habitat. This close relationship helps fulfill our inherent need to nurture. In the last two hundred years, the industrialization, mechanization, and urbanization in Western society has fractured this bond, leading to the diminishing of nurturing opportunities and affectionate interaction between people and their natural surroundings.

At no time in history have so many members of Western society been lacking in healthy interactions among themselves and with the environment. More people are electing to live alone, and many who are married choose not to have children. Singles or couples with children are compartmentalized. Many fathers and mothers work outside the home, usually in different locations and sometimes on different schedules. The children are usually born in a hospital, spend a lot of time in day care centers, and proceed to kindergarten, then elementary school and high school—usually all in different locations. When at home, the children are watching television or wearing headphones attached to a source of sound, usually loud music. Many children have little access to their grandparents.

Today's lack of nurturing opportunities and its compartmentalized lifestyle have resulted in increased stress, depression, loneliness, and other serious assaults on the health and well-being of a significant segment of our population. This situation presents many challenges to our health care professions, as well as opportunities for research, service, and teaching directed toward the restoration of the health of our society.

Those of us who explore the interaction of people, animals, and the natural environment cannot overestimate the significance of animals in the lives of the majority of our society. Companion animals defy compartmentalization and serve as nurturers for many people. They are also objects of nurture in that they promote touching, playing, and sharing with no time restraints.

The number of animals in the United States is impressive. Fifty-six percent of our 88 million households own over 220 million cats, dogs, birds, and other small animals. Over 100 million of these are cats and dogs. Animals (or their images) appear often in art, comics, celebrations, dreams, fables, folklore, food, imagination, language, medicine, music, photographs, religion, wishes, work, and worries. At long last, the importance of animals seems to be gaining recognition among more members of the health care professions.

In this chapter, I discuss recent observations that contribute to a better understanding of the interaction of people, animals, and our environment and how that understanding can be applied to our mutual benefit. I emphasize the human–animal interaction for the old and/or disabled. Finally, I review the contributions of the veterinary profession and suggest further promising areas of investigation.

Historical Perspective on Animal-Assisted Therapy

Primitive people found that people–animal partnerships were important to their well-being, if not vital to their survival. Many of Earth's early inhabitants formed a strong alliance, sometimes a symbiotic, or mutually dependent, relationship with animals. The most noteworthy relationship was with the dog; perhaps the very first was men and dogs hunting together in a mutual assistance pact. When dogs were domesticated, each became dependent on the other; probably neither could have survived alone. Undoubtedly, it would have been far more difficult for men to hunt other animals for food without the dogs' scent-tracking and attack capabilities.

Early people often worshiped, or at least recognized, beasts as special. They looked at animals as possessing cunning, courage, healing potential, and a power beyond human power. Because they thought these beasts understood human language, they communicated with them. Early people talked very seriously to animals and asked pardon when it was their painful duty to hunt and kill them.

The sense of an absolute distinction or separation between human and beast so prevalent in our world was hardly to be found among the early earth dwellers. Religious interpretations and beliefs have contributed to this separation, as have philosophers such as René Descartes. The eighteenth-century French philosopher believed that animals were machines devoid of consciousness and souls, and lacking the ability to feel pleasure or pain. Unfortunately, Descartes's beliefs were incorporated into traditional nineteenth-century biology and medicine and are with us still, although there is increasing evidence that animals do have consciousness. Descartes's philosophy may, at least in part, explain why many members of our health delivery system do not regard companion animals as significant others, even though most patients own pets.

The history of the use of animals as "therapeutic facilitators" for improving the health and well-being of people is interesting but has not been systematically studied or documented. It is only in the last forty years that articles on the health benefits of animals have been published in journals, and most have appeared in the last two decades. It is impossible to determine when animals were first used to promote the physical and psychological well-being of people, but animals and parts of animals have been used by healers throughout history. The pharmacopoeia of almost every nation referred to the use of various parts of animals in therapy. The cat was thought by many ancients to possess supernatural powers. Dogs, too, occupied an esteemed place on the healing team. Recent evidence suggests that dogs were companions for humans possibly before their use in hunting or as guardians. In ancient Greece, dogs were used to lick patients to promote healing. History is replete with the involvement of animals in remarkable preventive and therapeutic measures for an assortment of conditions.

In 1859, Florence Nightingale noted that "a small pet is an excellent companion for the sick. A pet bird in a cage is sometimes the only pleasure of an invalid confined to the same room for years."[1]

The use of horseback riding for individuals with disabilities has appeared in the literature for centuries. The Greeks, perhaps as early as 500 B.C., gave horseback rides to individuals considered untreatable or incurable in order to improve their spirits.

Bain reviewed the medical literature of the eighteenth and nineteenth centuries and found several references to the use and benefits of horseback riding. Reide noted that early reference was also made to the appropriateness of a "newly discovered" type of movement: the three-dimensional motion of a horse. The first study of the value of horseback riding was undertaken by Chassigne in Paris in 1875. He observed that riding was most beneficial in the treatment of hemiplegia, paraplegia, and other neurological disorders. Specifically, he noted an improvement in posture, balance, joint movement, and muscle control, which he ascribed to the active and passive movements provided by the horse. Recent observations confirm these benefits.

An interesting development involving horseback riding is hippotherapy, literally, "help of the horse." Although it has been used in Germany for some time, orthopedists in North America are now becoming interested in the therapy and are promoting its use. Specially trained physical and occupational therapists use this medical treatment for patients with movement disorders.

In hippotherapy, the therapist positions the patient on the horse. During treatment, the therapist analyzes the patient's responses to the horse's movements and directs the movement of the horse accordingly. The goal of hippotherapy is to improve the patient's posture, coordination, balance, mobility, and function.

The first use of animals in a U.S. hospital probably occurred in 1919. Secretary of the Interior Franklin K. Lane wrote to W. A. White, Superintendent of St. Elizabeth's Hospital in Washington, D.C., and suggested that dogs be introduced for the men to "play and chum with." As Dr. White supported the idea, it is assumed that dogs were introduced, though recorded results have not come to light.[2]

The second known use of animals in therapy in the United States occurred in the 1940s at an Army Air Corps convalescent hospital in Pawling, New York. The Pawling Center received Air Corps personnel from every theater of operations during World War II. The patients, convalescing from injuries or recovering from the effects of operational fatigue, were deemed to need a regime of restful activity. An academic program was designed to keep their minds active and, at the same time, give them surcease from war and its activities. The patients were encouraged to work at the center's farm with hogs, cattle, horses, and poultry. They also benefited from the "healing powers" of snakes, frogs, turtles, and other living creatures of the field and forest, as well as from the fields and forests themselves.[3] The experiment was considered successful, but it was stopped in a cost-saving move.

After World War II, some modest efforts were directed toward using companion animals in therapy. Boris Levinson, a clinical psychologist at Yeshiva University in New York City, discovered the great advantages of companion animals in therapy and promoted their use in many situations. He called for systematic and rigorous research to study their effectiveness, at the same time cautioning that we must learn how to select and train animals for special psychotherapeutic work.

Sam and Elizabeth Corson and their associates took up Levinson's charge at Ohio State University, where they were among the first to attempt, systematically, to evaluate pet-facilitated therapy. The Corsons introduced pets to patients who had failed to respond to so-called standard therapy (e.g., drugs and electroshock). They attempted to match the temperaments of the dogs with the needs of special patients. The results of the Corsons' experiments were very encouraging. Some patients who had been bedridden and uncommunicative were helped and eventually discharged. The Corsons reasoned that the pets were effective in psychotherapy because, to a withdrawn individual, they were undemanding, uncritical friends that served as loving links for those who had lost social skills and desires. Further, the pets needed to be fed, bathed, and brushed. As the patients assumed these nurturing duties, the Corsons noted that they began taking better care of themselves.

Animals in Institutions

There are countless animal interaction programs for people who are elderly, disabled, hospitalized, and/or incarcerated. Most of these programs are for people who are elderly and residing in institutions. Some of these programs have been under way for a long time, but the past decade has seen a rapid proliferation of such programs. Although the effects of these programs, which involve a variety of subjects in differing conditions, have been documented, the majority of the early reports had little or no scientific basis. All the same, most of the results seemed to be positive.

The most complete review of this subject was presented by Susanne Robb at a 1987 technical assessment workshop at the

National Institutes of Health. For her review, Robb selected twenty-five studies involving animal interaction with the elderly in long-term-care facilities. Group sizes varied from 3 to 104, the average being 30. When all of these studies were combined and examined, a number of health benefits were confirmed.

Interaction with companion animals made the residents smile and talk more, reach out toward people and objects, exhibit more alertness and attentiveness, and experience more well-being, higher morale, and/or greater satisfaction. Lower levels of depression were also observed. It was also noted that, when animals were present, older people manifesting cognitive impairments became less aggressive or agitated, were less insistent on occupying certain areas, and were less bizarre in their verbalizations.

When tested against alternative therapies, companion animals were superior in producing psychosocial benefits to arts and crafts, stuffed (plush) pets and videotapes depicting pets, or visitors. Several recent studies substantiate some of these observations, for example, the advantage of a visit by a pet and person over a person visiting alone.

Dr. Robb's views after her exhaustive study are interesting indeed:

> We know more about health benefits of pets for elderly people than we knew about other therapies that began with less debate. The drug lithium chloride was approved as safe and effective for treating bipolar disorder. For no apparent reason, psychiatrists used the drug for other forms of depression. Some of these people benefited clinically and were apparently not harmed. Coronary bypass surgery and total mastectomies were widely used before their efficacy was tested. Alternative therapies were not considered. No cost-benefit ratios were determined. No endorsements were required from clients or staff to implement them.
>
> Regarding pets as therapy for elderly people, enough research-based information has been produced to proceed with policy and program development. With reasonable attention to animal selection, problems of zoonoses (diseases communicable to humans from other animals) and injuries have not materialized. Animals seem to tolerate the

> work without ill effects. While all residents do not benefit, no harm accrues to those who do not.[4]

The exception would be a resident with a serious allergy. A study of 284 nursing homes over a period of one year found no pet-related allergies and observed that, for the residents, pets were safer than people in terms of infection and accident risk. A concern recently surfaced about people who have had their spleens removed. The U.S. Armed Forces Epidemiological Board recommended that those splenectomized individuals who own pets should be advised of the hazard of serious infections from a bacteria that may follow bites by cats and dogs.[5]

Though many people agree that animal interaction with humans is both psychologically and socially beneficial, they question the practicality of this intervention; administrators want to know if it is cost-effective. In this regard, I found the studies of Judith Siegel of special interest. She studied the effect of pet ownership and psychological distress on the use of physicians by 938 Medicare enrollees in a health maintenance organization. She found that the respondents who owned pets reported fewer physician contacts over the one-year period than the respondents who did not own pets. The pets seemed to help their owners in times of stress. Dog owners, particularly, seemed buffered from the impact of stressful life events. Dr. Siegel observed that dog owners, in comparison to owners of other pets, spent more time with their pet and felt that their pet was more important to them. Dogs, more than other pets, provided their owners with companionship and an object of attachment. There were indications that both psychological distress and not owning a pet were related to higher levels of illness behavior. Dr. Siegel's data support the notion that the promotion of pet ownership may reduce the demand for care for medically nonserious problems.

Many veterinarians have been particularly active and innovative in developing and implementing animal interaction programs in institutions. I give here just a few examples of the valuable work being done by veterinarians in this area.

In Washington, D.C., veterinarian Earl Strimple initiated an animal visitation and placement program in nursing and convalescent homes (including St. Elizabeth's Hospital) and in a federal prison.

Jean Hawkins, working with a nurse in Boise, Idaho, developed a children–pet visitation program in a local nursing home. They brought latchkey children, as well as Girl Scouts and 4-H members, into a veterinary clinic to teach them about animals and animal medicine. In order to prepare them for visiting elderly people, these workers taped the hands of the children, put cotton in their ears, and gave them dark glasses to wear. In this "handicapped" state, the children were asked to perform such tasks as opening pillboxes, reading signs, and conversing. This program has been very instructive and rewarding for the children and beneficial to the residents of the nursing home. Most of the elderly seem to enjoy the children and animal visitors more than any other activity.

Patrick Ryan is a public health veterinarian who is director of comparative medical and veterinary services in the Los Angeles County Department of Health Services. He has initiated a very interesting pet visitation and resident animal program at Rancho Los Amigos Medical Center, a county long-term-care facility for adults and children with severe physical disabilities, many of whom will spend the rest of their lives in a hospital. The center is affiliated with the University of Southern California School of Medicine. Ryan and his associates have developed an evaluative program of the effects of pet visitation on the health and well-being of severely disabled people.

Veterinarian Jim Dorn, impressed with what he had heard about the benefits of animals, volunteered to help start a pet visitation program with memory-disordered residents in the Florida Manor. The program involved working with faculty of the University of Central Florida College of Health to develop a protocol that would contribute to a data base measuring the effectiveness of pet visitation on patients with Alzheimer's disease. Dr. Dorn has brought much joy and happiness to the residents, probably restoring a degree of the ability to reminisce, recollect experiences, or share memories to seriously affected people, who are often forgotten or ignored by their families. The ability to reminisce may benefit health.

Animals in Hospitals

Although most human–animal interaction programs are carried out in institutions for the elderly, some of the most interesting and challenging occur in hospitals, including general-service, psychiatric, head-trauma, military, veterans', rehabilitation, acute-care, substance-abuse, long-term-care, neurology, geriatric, and AIDS hospitals. The stated purposes of visiting or resident animals in hospitals are socialization by friendly visitors, initiating communication, security, contact comfort (e.g., during dialysis or other unpleasant procedures), distraction, play, fun and laughter, minimizing pain, combating loneliness, nurturing, teaching tricks, riding (as on ponies), and education.

The prescription pet program at the Children's Hospital in Denver, Colorado, is a premier one and a good model for other hospitals. It began with the efforts of two veterinarians, Jan Facinelli and James Houchens, and a hospital administrator, Fern Bechtel, who, in 1983, began planning the program. Physicians and other health professionals, along with the Denver area Veterinary Medical Association and the Children's Hospital Medical Board, were also involved in the planning. In 1985, the program was officially implemented in the cancer ward.

Specially trained volunteers take their carefully screened dogs on a leash to patients selected by the physicians. A written parental and physician consent form is required for pet visitation. Visitation has now been extended to all wards (except the intensive-care and newborn wards); one specially screened team visits a locked psychiatric ward. The patient's nurse is present during the visit to supervise the volunteer. The program is periodically evaluated and monitored by medical professionals, veterinarians, and volunteer staff. (Information packets on animals in hospitals are available from the Delta Society, Box 1080, Renton, Washington 98057.)

The animal-assisted therapy program at the Baylor Institute for Rehabilitation in Dallas, Texas, is an excellent one for the elderly and/or disabled. This ninety-two-bed hospital incorporates the program into the therapy regimen for patients who have experienced strokes, traumatic brain injury, spinal cord injury, and other neurological and orthopedic conditions. Occupational therapist Shari Bernard, the full-time program coordinator, is assisted by over thirty volunteers and animals (principally dogs). A veterinarian helps her in the animal selection process, a long, tedious, and critical aspect of the program. Because of its success, a trial therapy program has been extended to the parent organization, the Baylor University Medical Center.

Guidelines for Animal Visitation and Placement

In order to address an assortment of problems associated with animal introduction into various institutions, we began forming components of the People-Pet-Partnership (PPP) in 1975. This program is a public service activity of Washington State University's College of Veterinary Medicine in conjunction with other departments and members of the community. (For information, contact the author, College of Veterinary Medicine, Bustad Hall 110, Washington State University, Pullman, Washington 99164-7010.)

The PPP supervises three community-oriented programs: (1) the Pet Education Partnership, which provides a curriculum on responsible animal care for preschool to sixth-grade children; (2) the Companion Animal Partnership (CAP), which explores and implements ways in which animals contribute to the well-being of people of all ages; this program includes the development of a prison partnership (i.e., a dog-training program at a maximum-security prison for women; and (3) the Partnership in Equine Therapy and Education (PETE), which offers classes for people who are disabled. All these programs depend on volunteers, including university students and members of the community.

Our People-Pet Partnership program receives many requests, such as for guidelines for establishing successful visiting and resident animal programs, including animal selection criteria for nursing homes and other institutions. Legislation in several states and at the federal level allowing animals in certain institutions has added urgency to these requests.

In response, members of the PPP and the Delta Society developed *Guidelines: Animals in Nursing Homes*, published by the California Veterinary Medical Association (CVMA) and revised in July 1987. (It is available from the Delta Society, Box 1080, Renton, Washington 98057; or the CVMA, 5231 Madison Avenue, Sacramento, California 95841). Selection procedures are discussed in the guidelines and also in a brochure entitled "The Veterinarian's Way of Selecting a Proper Pet," published by the American Veterinary Medical Association.

General response categories explained in the guidelines include dogs' responses to approach, handling, and interaction (play), as well as their sound sensitivity, pain threshold, manners, and responses to unexpected events.

I feel that animal selection is critical; the nature of the interaction and the strength of the bond that develops between people and animals depend in great part on the animal selected. Veterinarians must assume major responsibility in the selection process, also taking into account the animals' needs and well-being.

Animal Ownership in Rented Housing or Institutions

A federal law, passed in 1983, ensures the right of people who are elderly and/or handicapped living in government-assisted rental housing to own pets. Following is a partial excerpt from the law:

Pet Ownership in Assisted Rental Housing for the Elderly or Handicapped

Sec. 227.(1) No owner or manager of any federally assisted rental housing for the elderly or handicapped may

(1) as a condition of tenancy or otherwise, prohibit or prevent any tenant in such housing from owning common household pets or having common household pets living in the dwelling accommodations of such tenant in such housing; or

(2) restrict or discriminate against any person in connection with admission to, or occupancy of, such housing by reason of ownership of such

pets by, or the presence of such pets in the dwelling accommodations of, such person.[6]

Although administrators of governmentally assisted housing for elderly people voiced many concerns about the enactment of these laws (e.g., increased work load, personal injury, and property damage), a three-year experience in California showed that most concerns regarding permitting pets in these housing projects were unjustified. Most administrators, finding animal owners to be very responsible, rated the program as positive, and only 16 percent gave it a negative rating. Even non-pet-owners were positive, 69 percent favoring the law. Managers noted that, in general, the pet-owning residents felt more secure, had a more positive mental attitude, exercised more regularly, and had a more well-rounded life.

When a clearly written animal policy is established and enforced, very few problems arise. Successful management practices are based on addressing tenants' needs and communicating concerns.

Veterinarians have contributed and can and must contribute to successful placements by helping to establish appropriate guidelines and by helping in the selection of animals. They must also remain active in maintaining the health and well-being of the tenants' animals and in promoting obedience training.

Death and Grief

Animals are often intimately connected, in varied ways, with the processes of death and grief. Just as the death of a member of a client's family requires great sensitivity from veterinarians as well as society at large, so does the death of a companion animal. Though the euthanasia of an old or ill companion animal is frequent, it should never be taken lightly or become routine. No one should be surprised that many people mourn the loss of a companion animal as they mourn the loss of a child. Understandably, intense grief may accompany the diagnosis of terminal illness or the death of a dog, cat, or other companion animal. The situation may be further intensified if the owner depends on the animal as a guide dog or a hearing or assistance dog. This grief must be recognized and understood so that appropriate, enlightened, and compassionate treatment can be extended.

James Harris, a proponent of the human–animal bond for many years and chair of the American Veterinarian Medical Association Committee on the Human-Animal Bond, has been a very compassionate and effective communicator regarding grief. With special training in this area, he has raised the sensitivity of other veterinarians to the importance of addressing euthanasia, death, and grief.

More pet-loss support groups are needed to provide assistance to those who have lost or are about to lose a companion animal. The Animal Medical Center in New York is a leader in this effort. Director and veterinarian Bill Kay perceived the need and added social worker Susan Cohen to his staff. She counsels grieving clients and has formed a pet-loss support group.

More associations and individuals need to initiate and support such groups. In this regard, the Sacramento Valley Veterinary Medical Association sponsors such a group developed by the Human Animal Program at the University of California at Davis. This program has also established a pet-loss support hotline staffed by compassionate, trained volunteers, many of whom are veterinary students, whose education is greatly enhanced by this experience.

On an individual level, the combined efforts of veterinarian Rick Timmins and Don Marsh, whose companion animal had died, led to the formation of the support group Society for Animal Mourning. One of their activities is educating people in our society, who often frown on the display of grief at a pet's death. Such behavior causes the grieving person to feel uncomfortable about publicly expressing pain and sorrow.

At the other end of the spectrum, companion animals can help people who are terminally ill. The presence of a companion animal appears to reduce anxiety and to increase the comfort and adaptation of a terminally ill patient. Animals seem to provide a different kind of help and support than people do. In fact, people are often uncomfortable with terminally ill patients, avoiding contact whenever possible. When they are with these patients, they may dwell on their own concerns about death or may try to deter these patients from coming to terms with their final experience. Animals, conversely, are accepting; they do not shy away from a terminally ill patient but are very attentive.

Irene Muschel discussed the beneficial effects that animals have on the emotional well-being of terminally ill cancer patients. She observed that animal contact alleviated feelings of unhappiness and despair. Association with animals also helped these patients come to terms with their mortality.

A final point on the subject of grief concerns animals themselves. We must be aware that animals manifest the same signs of grief that people do. Their distress over loss or separation may compromise their health and well-being to the extent of being life-threatening.

Research on the Human–Animal Bond

Recently, impressive progress has been made in research on the human–animal bond. Some of the most striking research related to human–animal interaction has to do with physiological responses. Many people have observed the calming effect associated with a friendly creature that is furred, feathered, or finned. To test these observations, Aaron Katcher and his associates at the University of Pennsylvania examined the influence of human and nonhuman companionship on patients with severe coronary artery disease. Earlier, Erika Friedmann, when a graduate student with Dr. Katcher, along with other associates from the university, reported that patients with companion animals had better one-year survival rates than similar patients without animals.

Katcher and his associates pursued the influence of animal contact, especially touch and talk intimacy, on decreasing levels of arousal of the sympathetic nervous system and decreasing muscular tension. The researchers found that blood pressure was reduced when people touched and/or talked to animals. Friedmann reported at the 1987 National Institutes of Health

Technology Assessment workshop that, in a study of college students, the presence of animals modified the cardiovascular response (both heart rate and blood pressure) to a mild stressor by coronary-prone and non-coronary-prone individuals. Both groups benefited from the presence of an animal. This effect may go back to our early history, when we and other animals learned that the presence of calm animals indicated the absence of dangerous predators. These early observations by Katcher and his associates have been confirmed and extended by several investigators.

Poresky and others have observed that pet bonding, rather than pet ownership, is the critical determinant of the beneficial effects of animal association. He and his associates selected eight behaviors in order to develop a reliable companion-animal bonding scale. The scale induces questions such as: How often were you responsible for your companion animal's care? How often did you hold, stroke, or pet your companion animal? How often did you sleep near your companion animal? Using this scale, these researchers found that animal ownership was not a meaningful criterion for a beneficial human–animal association. In fact, the relationship can be detrimental to the health of both the animal and the owner if the association is negative.

The presence of animals may bring about consistent changes in speech patterns and facial expression. Katcher, Beck, and their associates have spent many years measuring physiological responses in people's interactions with animals. Their observations on human and animal behavior have included vocal expression, in both natural and experimental settings, and an analysis of photographs taken by pet owners or other family members interacting with family pets.

Katcher *et al.* noted that, when talking to a pet, the person's voice became softer and had a higher pitch, and the facial expression was more relaxed, the lips frequently open and slightly pursed—often forming a smile. The speech pattern was broken into a small series of words, usually phrased as a question. Often the question was answered by the speaker.

Animal association may also

- Promote appropriate social behaviors in mentally impaired institutionalized elderly.
- Help patients (e.g., cancer patients) work through their anxiety and despair and reduce the sense of loneliness and helplessness that was evident when the patients were alone or preoccupied by their illness.
- Contribute to better adjustment and social skills.
- Enhance the psychological well-being of many individuals.

In order to gain understanding as well as legitimacy regarding the health benefits of animal association, more extensive research must be done. The nature of human–animal bonding itself has yet to be determined.

Contributions of Veterinarians to Human–Animal Bond Programs

Many veterinarians and associates have realized great satisfaction in developing service programs involving the introduction of animals into a wide array of situations, addressing the results of human–animal interactions in the media, or promoting teaching, service, and research on those interactions. Having noted the contributions of a few of my colleagues in institutional settings, I now demonstrate the diversity of other contributions by describing the activities of a few veterinarians and their associates. (I apologize for leaving out many outstanding contributors.) I hope that the wide range of nurturing activities mentioned will stimulate more people to initiate worthwhile programs for the mutual benefit of people and animals.

Ronald Anderson, Andrew Edney, and Bruce Fogle, veterinarians in England, were pioneers in work on the human–animal bond and encouraged an exchange of information at conferences; the first meeting on this subject with an international flavor was held under the auspices of the British Small Animal Veterinary Association (BSAVA) in 1974. In 1980, Dr. Edney opened the second conference sponsored by the BSAVA on "The Human-Companion Animal Bond," which Dr. Bruce Fogle chaired.

Bruce Fogle, a Canadian-trained veterinarian who has a very successful practice in London, has been a leader in the promotion of the human–animal bond in the United Kingdom and internationally. With Lady Barbara Wright, he started the hearing-dog program in England. He has contributed remarkably to the understanding of the human–animal bond through his popular and widely acclaimed books *Pets and Their People* and *Games Pets Play,* as well as the book he edited, *Interrelations between People and Pets.*

Veterinarian Mary Stewart at the Glasgow Veterinary School has been a long-time proponent of animal-facilitated therapy. She has investigated students' attitudes toward animals and the results of fracturing the bond between people and animals. She understands grief following the loss of a family member and the loss of pets, contributing to our knowledge in this critical area. I have assisted her in consultation for the Prince and Princess of Wales Hospice, where we support plans for a wing that will permit terminally ill patients to bring their companion animals to the hospice with them.

William McCulloch is a U.S. pioneer in the human–animal bond "movement." In the late 1960s, after reading Boris Levinson's books, he became engaged in activities associated with the promotion of human–companion-animal interaction. In 1968, he stated, "We must understand the effect of man the 'invader,' his technology, and his impact on man-animal relationships."[7]

McCulloch interested his associate Richard Dorn and his public-health graduate-school mentors, R. K. Anderson and Stan Diesch, in the implications of the "bond" for the veterinary profession. They and his younger brother, Michael McCulloch, a psychiatrist, teamed up to form the Delta Foundation (to be discussed in the next section) in the mid-1970s to promote investigations into human–animal interaction. William McCulloch was also the first chairman of the American Veterinary Medical Association Committee on the Human-Animal Bond.

In the 1970s, Drs. Anderson, Diesch, and Joe Quigley went on to develop the University of Minnesota Center to Study

Human-Animal Relationships and Environments (CENSHARE). Many universities now have centers devoted to this activity.

Dean Franklin Loew was an early contributor to research on the human–animal bond and has continued his interest and concern with the establishment of a Center for Animals at Tufts University School of Veterinary Medicine.

Charles Doney, a veterinarian in Seattle who had known much personal adversity in his life, conducted weekly free clinics for "street people" and low-income elderly. These people, to whom their animals are very meaningful, have no resources. Without Dr. Doney's services, their animals would have received no medical attention. Stan Coe and about a dozen other veterinarians volunteered to carry on his work after he died. Members of the Puget Sound Delta Society Chapter also assist in this effort.

These are only a few examples of the many notable activities of veterinarians. We wish we could report on all of the noteworthy contributions of veterinarians throughout the world. We must express gratitude to the many veterinarians who have volunteered their time to attend to animals in placements and/or animal programs in prisons, nursing and convalescent homes, hospitals, humane societies, and assistance-dog programs, and to the many veterinarians who truly understand the significance of the human–animal bond and apply their understanding of it in their daily practice, thereby fulfilling their responsibilities to both the patient and the client.

Delta Society and Other Organizations

Many organizations address the various facets of human–animal interactions. The first organization to address this "bond" was the Delta Foundation, formed in 1976 by a small group of veterinarians in the United States. It was concerned principally with research and educational needs.

In 1979, a meeting was held in Scotland to organize the first membership organization. Called the Group for the Study of the Human-Animal Bond (GSHAB), the original thirteen members included veterinarians and physicians, two of them from the United States. To accomplish growth and outreach and encourage the needed research, we in the United States formed a membership organization, the Delta Society, with close ties to the GSHAB (now called the Society for Companion Animal Studies—SCAS). The Delta Society developed from the Delta Foundation in 1981 and established offices in the Greater Seattle area in 1983.

The leading international resource on the interactions of people, animals, and the environment, the Delta Society offers information on:

- Worldwide pet-facilitated therapy programs and the leaders in the human–animal bond field.
- Guidelines for starting effective animal programs in local communities, nursing homes, prisons, hospitals, and other institutions.
- Current and past research describing the effect of animals on people's health and well-being.
- Audiovisual and educational materials.
- Legislation and procedures that allow companion animals in housing complexes and institutions.

The society sponsors or cosponsors national (annual) and international (triennial) conferences that include both scientific sessions and workshops. It hosted an international conference in Boston in 1986 attended by over one thousand people from sixteen countries. Delta also publishes a membership magazine called *People-Animals-Environment*. *Anthrozoos: The Journal of the Delta Society,* edited by Andrew Rowan of Tufts University, is published quarterly and presents scientific findings regarding human–animal interactions. (For information, contact Linda Hines, Executive Director, Box 1080, Renton, Washington 98057.)

Delta Australia was formed recently under the leadership of veterinarian Roger Lavelle and his associates. The Joint Advisory Committee on Pets in Society was founded earlier by the late veterinarian Stirling Hogarth-Scott and his associates.

The French organization is L'Association Francaise d'Information et de Recherche sur l'Animal de Compagnie (AFIRAC).

AFIRAC, with the cosponsorship of the Delta Society and various national societies, held an international conference on human–animal interactions in Monte Carlo in November 1989, attended by over six hundred people from twenty-five countries.

The Austrian Society is called the Institute for Interdisciplinary Research on the Human-Pet Relationship (IEMT). It organized an outstanding international symposium in 1983 entitled "The Human-Pet Relationship" to honor Nobel Laureate Konrad Lorenz on his eightieth birthday. Following this meeting, the Human-Animal Contact Study Group was formed in South Africa.

There is growing interest in establishing societies in Italy, Belgium, and Japan. Canadians have recently formed the Human Animal Bond of Canada (HABAC).

Recommendations for Future Contributions

Following are some ways in which veterinarians can contribute their knowledge and expertise to other professionals and to the public at large:

1. Provide professional counsel regarding noninfectious diseases, animal temperament and selection criteria, and the prevention of zoonotic diseases (those that are transferred from animals to people), including vaccination schedules for candidate companion animals for placement in animal-assisted therapy programs.
2. Become better informed about animal behavior and its modification. A better understanding of human behavior is also a vital area for study and improved understanding.
3. Inculcate in all people a greater reverence for life.
4. Serve as a resource for disabled people by recommending training programs, sources of assistance animals, or other resources involving animals that may be helpful.

5. Learn to deal in a comfortable and comforting way with people who are disabled, most especially those who are strongly bonded with an assistance animal on whom their freedom and independence rest.
6. Develop, working with other professionals, new and innovative measures to enable more people who are elderly, lonely, disabled, and poor to obtain, maintain, and provide for companion animals.
7. Assist in organizing members of local humane, youth, and other groups to take animals for regular visits to area nursing homes and other institutions.
8. Encourage hospitals and hospices to have assigned wards where patients who request their animals to accompany them will be accommodated. Urge hospitals to include on admissions forms questions such as: Do you live alone? Do you have pets? Who should be called to take care of them?
9. Assist in establishing reasonable legislation, rules, guidelines, and procedures for allowing animals in institutions and public housing.
10. Establish disaster plans in all critical areas that include provisions for the evacuation and care of animals as well as people.
11. Recommend at least two companion animals of different ages rather than only one in a household, especially for people who are elderly and disabled as well as single persons.
12. Help implement animal programs in penal institutions and encourage investigations regarding the ability of some prisoner-trained dogs to detect seizures in people before the person is aware of an impending seizure.
13. Improve and expand training for veterinarians, animal technicians, and more of our social workers and health care professionals in grief counseling for those who have suffered the loss of animals with which they were closely bonded. Encourage more groups to form regularly scheduled grief counseling sessions.
14. Support increased data-based research pertaining to

human–animal interaction and animal-assisted therapy. If animal-assisted therapy offers hope for relief of human suffering and also benefits the animals involved, it is our professional obligation to explore every avenue for its use.

15. Encourage research efforts on and participate in service for patients suffering from Alzheimer's disease, the fourth leading cause of death in the United States. Veterinarians James Dorn, Gamal Zaki, and others have observed that companion animal intervention causes many positive behavioral changes in patients, including increased socialization, better coping and communications skills, and increased reminiscence and physical activity. Such interventions also have a calming effect.
16. Future national health surveys should include questions related to the presence or absence of closely bonded animals (including questions that clearly define the nature of the bonding), as studies suggest a link between closely bonded companion animals and the long-term health and well-being of people. Also, the existing large epidemiological studies should be reexamined, and follow-up data should be obtained on any link of disease incidence (e.g., cardiovascular disease) and the presence or absence of a closely bonded animal.
17. Conjointly with other experts, establish criteria for the certification of all classifications of assistance animals, as well as animal-assisted therapists and animal trainers.
18. Promote programs that train certified assistance animals.
19. Develop a strategy to obtain third-party payment for animal-assisted therapy.

Notes

1. C. W. Smith, *Florence Nightingale*. New York: McGraw-Hill, 1951.
2. T. Wolfle and R. Whitney, personal communication, 1987.

3. Ed Menning, personal communication, 1979.
4. S. S. Robb, *Summary of Health Benefits of Pets for Elderly Residents in Health Care Centers,* presented at NIH Technology Assessment Workshop on Health Benefits of Pets, Bethesda, Maryland, September 10–11, 1987.
5. L. J. Anderson, personal communication, 1989.
6. *Congressional Record,* Vol. 129, No. 160—Part II, November 17, 1983.
7. William McCulloch, personal communication, 1968.

Suggested Reading

L. K. Bustad, "Recent Discoveries about Our Relationships with the Natural World," in *Compassion: Our Last Great Hope,* ed. L. K. Bustad. Renton, WA: Delta Society, 1990.

O. Cusach and E. Smith, *Pets and the Elderly: The Therapeutic Bond.* New York: Haworth Press, 1984.

A. H. Katcher and A. M. Beck (eds.), *New Perspectives on Our Lives with Companion Animals.* Philadelphia: University of Pennsylvania Press, 1983.

11

Psychology and the Mental Health Needs of the Elderly

GARY R. VANDENBOS, PH.D.

Introduction

There is considerable debate on the nature and extent of the psychological, behavioral, and mental health needs of the elderly. Their receptivity to acknowledging such problems and seeking psychological treatment and care is also being debated. All too often, such debates obscure or confuse the issues related to the mental health care of the elderly.

The sad fact is that the elderly are underserved by all current mental-health service-delivery systems and all current health-care funding mechanisms. Consequently, the mental health needs of the elderly simply are not being adequately met. In the mid-1980s, there were approximately 26 million individuals aged sixty-five or older, representing about 12 percent of the total U.S. population. Although rough estimates suggested that somewhere between 2.5 and 7.5 million individuals out of this elderly population had emotional and behavioral problems that were serious enough to warrant professional intervention, the most solid national estimate set the figure at 19 percent of the elderly population, or 5 million individuals.

A number of factors seem to contribute to the underutilization of mental health services among the elderly. It has been fashionable to talk about the anti-mental-health bias within the current elderly population. There is no question that today's elderly are less psychologically sophisticated and less psychologically oriented than younger age groups. However, this pattern is changing.

Other reasons for the low utilization of mental health services by the elderly include misinformation about the nature and value of psychological care; lack of knowledge about the availability of services; inaccessibility due to a general lack of integrated support services (e.g., outreach, home visits, and transportation); the intimidating regulations and paperwork required for mental-health insurance benefits; bias among mental health providers regarding the elderly; and financial, language, and cultural barriers in the case of elderly minorities.

Until very recently, major biases within the funding mechanisms have made it difficult for the elderly to seek psychological help. These include the artificial cap on mental-health-services funding under Medicare and the ineligibility for reimbursement of psychologists and other nonphysician mental-health professionals by this program. These regulations have been amended recently, so the pattern of underutilization may soon change.

Psychology has much to contribute to health care for the elderly, including prevention, clinical intervention, and basic care. My comments focus on four aspects of this premise. First, I discuss the kinds of mental-health-care problems about which the elderly see psychologists. Second, I examine how the elderly come in contact with psychologists. Third, I briefly mention where psychologists see and treat elderly patients. Finally, I discuss the kinds of clinical services provided by psychologists to elderly patients, as well as the life span assessment and the three most common mental-health problems of elderly patients.

Why Older Individuals See Psychologists

The problems for which older individuals see psychologists are mostly similar to those of any other age group within the general U.S. population. The elderly, as a group, are generally found to have slightly fewer mental-health problems of all types, with the exception of dementia.

The major mental-health problems among the elderly include depression and other mood disorders; dementia and severe cognitive impairment; suicide (particularly among men over seventy-five); alcohol abuse; polydrug use and misuse of prescription medications; and chronic mental disability. Such problems frequently involve problem behavior, memory problems, and strained family and social relations.

The two most frequent problems about which an elderly patient sees a psychologist are (1) concern related to memory problems and (2) some vague awareness that "I'm not feeling very good." Both are relatively nonspecific complaints. Thoughtful and comprehensive clinical assessments are clearly necessary.

In the first instance, the patient may or may not have a memory problem. A careful clinical assessment accurately assesses memory and cognitive functioning. Among other things, it also determines whether depression exists, identifies the side effects of medications, explores possible alcohol abuse, and examines relationship dynamics, all of which can affect memory and cognition.

Initially, the psychologist should consider potentially reversible processes that may be producing or exacerbating the cognitive symptoms and should then assess and treat them when appropriate. Such symptoms may be due to the side effects of drugs, malnutrition, metabolic and endocrine disorders, infectious diseases, and brain tumors.

Next, irreversible but nonprogressive brain damage, such as head trauma or strokes, should be considered and differentiated from progressive disorders.

Finally, relying largely on history and medical features, the psychologist should differentiate Alzheimer's disease from multi-infarct dementia (MID), which is stroke- or heart-attack-related, or other progressive dementias. Repeated testing and assessment over time constitute the best way of diagnosing dementia. If a diagnosis of Alzheimer's disease is eventually made, it is almost always made by first excluding all other causes of the symptoms.

For the patient who isn't "feeling good," a thorough clinical assessment is also needed. Inevitably, such elderly patients have been seen or are seeing one or more physicians; a lack of medical contact or screening is rarely the problem. Rather, it is either that no physiological basis for the problem has been found, or that some physical problem is being treated but the more generalized problem of "not feeling good" persists.

The psychological assessment explores such areas as health status and physical health treatments; prescription and nonprescription drug use (and the side effects or interactive effects of medication); mental health status (depression, anxiety, etc.); social and family changes (and factors such as financial difficulties or unresolved grief); control issues in family relations; and the psychological reaction to normal physical aging.

How Older Individuals Contact Psychologists

Elderly patients come into contact with psychologists through direct self-initiated contact, through organized-care systems, and through referrals by other health professionals, just as do all other patient groups seen by psychologists.

Psychologists are frequently the first point of contact for mental health care of the elderly; there is not a formal referral by a physician. Such direct initial contacts probably account for almost 50 percent of the contacts between elderly patients and psychologists.

In such direct-contact situations, the elderly individual or the family are concerned about specific behaviors or symptoms that they view as psychological, not physical, problems. Inevitably, the patient is already receiving competent medical care, so collaboration, not formal referral, is all that is necessary. Some of these patient-initiated visits occur because the elderly patient or the family have been unsuccessful in getting the physician to address a specific concern, or because of an adverse effect of some medical intervention. For example, the patient or family may be concerned about a newly emerged memory problem that seemingly developed after the patient started on a new medication, or the patient may be concerned about a combination of weight increase, general fatigue, and early-evening drowsiness. These symptoms may be related to medication change, depression, or other factors.

Referrals by general-practice physicians or general-practice nurses probably account for another 35 to 40 percent of elderly patient contacts with psychologists. For those physicians and nurses who appropriately identify emotional and behavioral problems in the elderly and make referrals, psychologists are frequently the mental health provider of choice.

The third most frequent way in which elderly patients come to psychologists is through organized-care systems. That is, the contact may be stimulated by a social worker or other professional in a community program, a health maintenance organization, a nursing home, a senior center, adult day care, a social service agency, or the courts.

Where Older Individuals See Psychologists

Until now, the most frequent site of service delivery by psychologists to elderly patients has been in organized-care settings. The Veterans Administration (VA) inpatient and outpatient programs makes extensive use of psychologists. Also, psychologists often provide care through outpatient clinics attached to general medical hospitals and health-care service centers. Elderly patients also see psychologists through community mental-health centers (CMHCs), although they use CMHC services proportionally less than the general population.

Community-based programs, such as area agencies on aging, senior centers, adult day-care centers, and "board-and-care" homes, provide still another venue where the elderly are likely to have contact with a psychologist. Social services departments may operate programs through which brief psychological consultation or information is provided, or contact may be stimulated by or provided through court-based intervention programs.

Contact with psychologists through nursing homes is still somewhat infrequent because of previous Medicaid restrictions, but it is likely to increase in light of recent legislative changes. On occasion, a psychologist is the primary therapist for an elderly patient in a private psychiatric hospital.

The provision of psychological services to elderly patients by private-practice psychologists is a small but significant source of contact. In 1989, the first session of the 101st Congress approved direct reimbursement for the professional services of psychologists under Part B of Medicare as a provision of the Omnibus Budget Reconciliation Act of 1989 (P.L. 101-239). With this new provision, such contact is likely to increase greatly in the coming years, thus ensuring the elderly access to needed psychological care.

Services Provided by Psychologists to Elderly Patients

Although definitive statistics do not exist, the most frequent service provided to elderly patients by psychologists is probably "assessment, referral, and linkage." The latter entails getting patients to the appropriate professionals, who then maintain a collaborative dialogue. Because of concerns about and problems with memory, assessment and psychological testing are used more frequently with elderly patients than with other adult populations. Such assessment and clinical interviews tend to be extensive, as it is often critical to interview the patient's spouse and family members in addition to the patient. Psychological testing is more frequent with elderly patients than with other adult populations both because of the nature of the referral and diagnostic questions, which are more complex for the elderly, and because of the need to make baseline assessments for future follow-up.

The second most frequent service provided by psychologists for elderly patients is clinical intervention and/or psychotherapy. The prognosis for elderly patients seen in psychotherapy is quite good. At least half of the psychotherapeutic interventions used with the elderly are short term, combining extended assessments with education and consultation. As with any other age group, this short-term psychotherapy most frequently focuses on a specific problem. This is *not* to say that the elderly are either unsuited to or do not benefit from longer term psychotherapy. They do. For some, formal psychotherapy is both effective and appropriate.

Family or couple work is somewhat more prevalent with other adult populations than with the elderly. The structure and process of such therapy may also be somewhat different for the elderly population. That is, by the time family therapy occurs, a fair amount of deterioration has usually taken place. Family work, then, is more likely to be similar to parent guidance sessions (as if one were treating a child), except that one is working with the adult children of the elderly patients or the higher functioning spouse. The sessions are more psychoeducational and skill building than psychotherapeutic and insight-oriented.

The third most frequent activity that psychologists provide to or on behalf of elderly patients is consultation with other professionals. Whether the initial referral of the patient to the psychologist came from another professional or was self-initiated by the older patient or by his or her family, the assessment will make it clear that consultation and collaborative planning with another professional are essential.

Life Span Assessment of Elderly Patients

Aging is a complex process involving a variety of patterns and a variety of ways of adapting. The accurate assessment of the elderly patient is a complex task, and there are few established guidelines for decision making. Existing test and assessment instruments may be helpful, but they are often inconclusive. In general, both clinical assessment and psychotherapy with elderly patients are more effective when the psychologist views, assesses, and treats the current problem by taking into account the patient's total current life circumstances and overall life history, that is, her or his life span assessment. Viewing problem behavior and psychological distress in older patients as isolated symptoms is clinically inefficient.

Adaptations in therapy for elderly patients are necessary

because of the developmental changes that come with aging; because of cohort effects, or those characteristics unique to a group of people who are all the same age at the same time and have lived through the same experiences together (e.g., today's elderly lived their formative adolescent years during the Great Depression); and because of changing social roles. At the same time, elderly patients must be understood as individuals within the context of their health, abilities, personal and social history, concept of self, and other variables. In short, clinicians must not lose sight of the usual goal of therapy: to understand the patient fully as a human being.

The therapist must consider several levels of concern in the psychological assessment of the elderly. The first level of concern about the elderly patient in therapy must deal with three general domains in which the problem may appear: physical illness, mood disturbance, and memory impairment. The second level of concern is how the problem manifests itself within each domain. The third level of concern, as mentioned above, should be understanding the patient as a person. Although therapy is generally problem-focused, the psychologist must realize that it is the person who has the problem, and a general understanding of that person's individuality is essential in directing the course of therapy.

It is helpful in therapy to have an understanding of the person's ethnic identity, values, religious background, family history (families in both childhood and in adulthood), work history, and past accomplishments. Understanding the whole person often leads to learning the patient's strengths and to a discovery of the solutions to his or her problems, such as a rediscovery of old skills.

Memory Assessment

Memory in older individuals serves as a sensitive barometer of physical and emotional well-being. Contrary to common belief, memory is not a single entity but a multidimensional process. This process includes the acquisition, the storage, and the retrieval of information and is influenced by the type of information (e.g., verbal, visual, or motor) to be remembered.

Although memory impairment is a major indicator of the dementia syndrome, memory problems occur in elderly patients for a variety of reasons. Mild memory loss is associated with the normal aging process and should be differentiated from the more pervasive, pathological changes that characterize dementia. Memory loss and other cognitive problems may also result from a wide range of illnesses, medications, and emotional disturbances.

A structured, comprehensive assessment of memory confirms both the presence and the type of memory impairment. The type and pattern of memory loss may suggest possibilities for rehabilitation or for planning care.

The assessment of memory in older patients can be approached in one of three ways: obtaining global ratings on general but limited tests, using comprehensive batteries of tests, or selecting individual tests for highly specific purposes. Each approach has different strengths and limitations. Tests that provide a global rating, such as mental status instruments like the Mini-Mental State Examination (MMSE), are most commonly used to assess memory. Such tests are used to determine orientation and the recall of simple information, and they sample a range of functions, such as attention, object recognition, drawing, writing, and following directions. Other global rating tests are used to assess the stage of a patient's dementia, as well as the cognitive and behavioral decline associated with Alzheimer's disease. The Dementia Rating Scale assesses five functions: attention, initiation and perseveration, construction, conceptualization, and memory. Although each test has some limitations in that each is unable to assess some dimension of memory, each nevertheless provides a broad profile of functioning that can be compared with nonimpaired functioning. What is probably ideal is for clinicians to develop a battery of tests to measure different memory functions and other key cognitive skills, such as language and spatial abilities. Individual tests can then be used selectively, depending on the patient's presenting problem.

There are various components of memory evaluation. A thorough clinical memory evaluation should have the following characteristics. The tests should be able to differentiate the acquisition of information from recall and should also measure delayed recall. The test battery should include a range of stimuli, using both verbal and nonverbal items. Some assessment of memory function in everyday situations must be made by obtaining specific information on the nature and the past and current history of the complaint of memory failure from the patient or the family. The degree to which a memory deficit disrupts a patient's everyday activities is an excellent indicator of the seriousness of the deficit. Subjective reports of memory loss may or may not correspond to objective performance assessments. Finally, as mentioned earlier, many factors affect memory: normal aging, a variety of illnesses, fatigue, depression or anxiety, hearing and vision impairments, level of education, and individual differences in ability.

Overall, when older patients express concern about memory problems, clinicians should treat their remarks as a serious statement of a real concern. If testing shows no memory problems, clinicians should explore other factors, such as family problems, that may be causing the concern.

Depression and Other Late-Onset Psychological Disorders

Depression is generally considered the most common mental-health problem in older individuals. Depression usually occurs following some major stressful event in the life of the older person, such as the loss of family members and friends or a major illness. However, in some cases, depression may occur for no readily apparent reason.

As in younger adults, depression in elderly patients may take many forms. It may range from adjustment reaction with depressed mood to a major depressive disorder accompanied by a sense of helplessness, guilt, loss of appetite, sleep disturbance, difficulty in concentrating, and thoughts of death and suicide. Depressed older persons may become unrealistically concerned about their memory, their thought processes (and content), and the idea of growing old (and that life is over). That is, they may worry that they are "suicidal" because they so often think about family and friends who are dead, think how much they miss them, and note that such thoughts are more frequent than when they were thirty years old. They worry that they are concentrating on death and dying when their thoughts really reflect their own aging, the real-world events around them, and normal reminiscence.

Studies do not show consistent support for the belief that depression increases with increasing age. Rather, in the view of some investigators, there is evidence that the elderly are relatively immune from depression, in contrast to young adults.

Differing conclusions about an age–depression relationship may be the result of different approaches to how depression is conceptualized and measured in various studies, coupled with other variations in research design and analysis. Two major types of measurement, with very different methodological approaches, have generally been used in research on depression and aging. These are the "standard-screening" measurement approach, which developed out of the psychometric tradition in psychology, and the "diagnostic-criteria" approach, which has its roots in psychiatry. Although these two methodological perspectives are based on a common conception of the depressive syndrome, they vary in their strategies of gathering, evaluating, and aggregating symptom data.

The approaches that have been used in the treatment of depression in older adults include behavioral therapy, cognitive therapy, interpersonal-focused therapy, psychodynamic approaches, and supportive therapy. In one variation of cognitive therapy, some clinicians used bibliotherapy in which a book, *Feeling Good* by David D. Burns, was read at home and discussed in sessions. Other research results have shown that cognitive and behavioral treatments were more effective with depressed individuals whose depression was triggered primarily by external events rather than by internal conflict.

Alcohol and Drug Assessment

In the conduct of most clinical evaluations of the elderly, it is important to consider the possible role and contribution of alcohol or drugs to the problems being experienced by the elderly patient. However, I wish to emphasize that these are two fairly different assessments.

The alcohol-related assessment is what one would typically expect, namely, a look at the frequency, quantity, and timing of alcohol consumption. However, by *drug assessment,* I do not mean an inquiry into the use of illegal drugs such as marijuana or cocaine. Illegal drug use among the current cohort of elderly is relatively low. Rather, I mean the unintended consequences and interaction effects of prescription drugs and over-the-counter medications. I will discuss the latter assessment first.

The clinical assessment of elderly patients should explore prescription *and* over-the-counter drug use. In most situations, this means specifically inquiring about and listing exactly what prescription and nonprescription medications the patient is taking, including how frequently and in what dosages. In some situations, it may be appropriate actually to have the patient bring in all medications so that they can be reviewed.

About two-thirds of the elderly population aged sixty and older take at least one over-the-counter medication daily for the treatment of one of the many age-related conditions (e.g., arthritis, constipation, and insomnia). Over-the-counter drug use increases with age, especially among females.

All too often, physicians prescribe medications to elderly patients without systematically reviewing what medications the patient is currently taking. Physicians also seem to prescribe medication to the elderly as if the medication will need to be taken forever, or the patient assumes this. It is not uncommon to find elderly patients taking eight, ten, or twelve different medications, half of which are no longer necessary. These practices can lead to toxicity and other types of adverse reactions. Elderly women are at a greater risk of physician-perpetuated drug abuse than any other group. Many of the so-called memory problems referred to psychologists turn out to be the result of the interaction effects or the cumulative toxic effects of multiple and chronic prescription and nonprescription drug use. The psychologist frequently needs to consult with the patient's primary physician to review the necessity of continuing various medications.

Some psychologists think that the organization of long-term-care institutions, specifically nursing homes, contributes significantly to drug abuse among the elderly. Because nursing homes generally lack skilled staff adequately trained in mental health care and in the handling of behaviorally disruptive elderly patients, there is a temptation to misuse drugs that have legitimate benefits to some patients, in order to maintain peace and order in the nursing home.

Relatively few elderly patients are referred to psychologists because of blatant alcohol abuse or alcoholism. However, alcohol problems among the elderly are more common than is generally recognized, and alcohol use should be assessed whenever the problem presented relates to depression, memory complaints, or conduct disorders. It is fairly common for elderly patients to attempt to treat emerging depression by the use of alcohol. Such efforts are generally unsuccessful, so that when clinicians see elderly patients, they frequently have at least two problems to treat.

Alcoholism is the second most frequent cause for admitting elderly patients to psychiatric hospitals. Estimates are that 80 percent of elderly patients taking an over-the-counter drug daily also use alcohol or prescription medications, or both. Elderly women are also at risk of self- and other-perpetuated abuse involving drug and alcohol interactions, as well as the abuse of legal psychotropics, such as Thorazine, Valium, and Prozac.

Research suggests that the older alcoholics and older substance abusers may come from distinct populations. Evidence indicates that older alcohol abusers had relatively stable early life patterns and began to experience alcohol problems in their forties and fifties. Older opiate abusers probably began in adolescence and then adopted a healthy lifestyle. Those who abused alcohol, barbiturates, tranquilizers, and other central nervous system depressants were frequently middle-class people who used these drugs most heavily between ages thirty and fifty.

Conclusion

The elderly, like other age cohorts, experience emotional and behavioral difficulties. These problems are eminently treatable when elderly patients are provided access to the appropriate care. When elderly patients have the means and financial mechanisms for access to psychologists, they use psychological services and benefit from them. Approximately half of such contacts are self-initiated, direct, initial clinical contacts. The recent changes in the Medicaid and Medicare laws will undoubtedly increase such contacts. As psychologists consider further changes in the nature and scope of their practice, including the possibility of limited prescription privileges, the range of their services to elderly patients will undoubtedly expand further.

Suggested Reading

Bob Knight, *Psychotherapy with Older Adults*. Beverly Hills, CA: Sage, 1986.

Leonard W. Poon (ed.), *Clinical Memory Assessment of Older Adults*. Washington, DC: American Psychological Association, 1986.

Martha Storandt and Gary R. VandenBos (eds.), *The Adult Years: Continuity and Change*. Washington, DC: American Psychological Association, 1989.

12

Psychiatric Health Care for the Elderly

ARNOLD M. LUDWIG, M.D.

Extent of the Problem

As the elderly population continues to increase over the next several decades, the problems of providing adequate health services will assume major proportions. The estimated number of U.S. citizens sixty-five or over is expected to jump from thirty-four million in 1995 to sixty-five million in 2030. That represents an increase from 13 percent of the population in 1995 to 21 percent in 2030.

Epidemiological studies, those that chart how much disease occurs and where in a population, indicate that the elderly have more mental health problems than any other age group. It is estimated that between 18 and 25 percent of the elderly have significant mental problems. Most are related to depression or impaired cognitive faculties; others pertain to anxiety, adjustment disorders, paranoid reactions, drug use, alcohol dependence, and a variety of other psychiatric conditions. Despite the magnitude of the problem, approximately 80 percent of those who needed psychiatric care in 1980 did not receive it. Further, only 2 percent of the Medicare dollar in 1979 was spent on mental health care for the elderly and disabled; this has not improved.

Growing public awareness of these trends has spurred significant developments in the aging area. Many more organizations at the local, state, and national levels have become actively involved in addressing the special mental health problems of the elderly.

In the psychiatric arena, two lead governmental agencies address a wide variety of issues: the National Institute on Aging and the Center on Aging at the National Institute for Mental Health. In 1980, the Mental Health System Act was designed to ensure comprehensive and coordinated mental health care for the elderly.

Despite these and other encouraging developments, many formidable problems remain, especially with regard to research, education, and treatment services for the rapidly expanding emotional needs of the aging, their families, and their communities.

Special Psychiatric Problems

The mental health problems of the aging population require special attention and expertise because, in many respects, they are different from those of other age groups. In this section, I discuss five major areas that affect and are affected by these problems.

Physical

As people age, they are likely to experience a progressively constricted sensory environment. Every sense is affected; that is, visual acuity tends to worsen, hearing becomes more impaired, the sense of smell lessens, taste diminishes, sensitivity to touch decreases, and balance and fine coordination are disturbed. These changes, which constitute a kind of sensory deprivation, make it more difficult for aging individuals to cope with many of the other common problems of growing old. Depression, anxiety, paranoia, anger, and fear often accompany these impaired perceptual functions.

Many elderly individuals also experience a decreased sense of vitality and an increased sense of debility or ill health. Other common changes include less capacity to enjoy sexual activity, impaired sexual performance, altered sleep patterns, and the diminished ability to sustain alertness. All of these impairments tend to undermine self-confidence and feelings of autonomy and independence.

Unfortunately, aging is also a time of serious and protracted illness. Many chronic diseases, such as hypertension, diabetes, intestinal malabsorption, diverticulitis, arthritis, emphysema, and a host of other nagging ailments, require major psychological adjustments. The medications used to treat these conditions often create problems in their own right, producing a number of undesirable side effects or deleterious drug interactions.

Cognitive Deficits

As people age, they are prone to a wide variety of cognitive deficits involving deficiencies in concentration, memory, and awareness. Besides minor reductions in short-term memory, often part of the normal aging process, major impairments in cognition may occur as part of various brain-deteriorating diseases, the most common being Alzheimer's disease and multi-infarct dementia, which involves a series of small blockages of brain tissue.

Other cognitive dysfunctions that tend to be associated with age are deficits in sustained attention, mental acuity, linguistic fluency, problem-solving ability, and abstraction. All diminish the capacity of elderly individuals to cope with the ordinary stresses of everyday living. Because depression in the elderly may also produce many of the same changes, the ability to distinguish depression and dementia is one of the greatest challenges of geriatric psychiatry. Some of the clinical signs of depression ("pseudodementia"), for example, include an awareness of failing memory, a history of prior emotional difficulties, excessive emphasis on disability, rapid mood changes, and an early deterioration in social skills.

Psychological Difficulties

It is an unfortunate paradox that many aging individuals with the fewest physical and cognitive resources for coping with difficulties are often exposed to the greatest number of life stresses: death of loved ones, relatives, and friends; moves to new residential settings; adjustments to unfamiliar surroundings; retirement; shrinking social networks; and forced isolation and loneliness.

Many other problems, both physical and psychic, compound these stresses, such as coming to grips with one's own mortality, increasing dependency, chronic pain, relative disability, and, in many instances, the humiliation of being unable to control bowel or bladder function or to take care of one's own personal hygiene. In addition to all these problems, older people are also increasingly vulnerable to attack, exploitation, and crime, especially in urban settings where they are less able to defend themselves or flee. It is not surprising to find a heightened prevalence of depression, anxiety, paranoid reactions, hypochondriasis, and increased drug and alcohol use among the elderly.

Social and Familial Networking

A progressively constricted social environment is apt to be a consequence of old age, as is a reduction in meaningful interactions with others. Further aggravating this situation is a growing inability on the part of the elderly to use adequate transportation or to drive themselves around town for visits because of increased incoordination, slowed reflexes, and impaired sight. These social stresses often have a particularly great impact on people who have worked all their lives and are not adequately prepared for retirement and the absence of productive work.

In addition, many elderly experience a progressive economic decline, a decreased standard of living, and a diminished sense of self-worth as their income stops and their retirement funds shrink in value. This process may become especially traumatic for those elderly who are forced to abandon their homes and relocate in nursing facilities or special housing units for the elderly.

Therapeutics

The problems of treating and managing the medical conditions of the elderly are complicated by a number of special considerations. First, many individuals are unable to make office visits to the doctor or the hospital for laboratory tests or diagnostic purposes because of their inability to drive or obtain adequate transportation.

One of the most common problems is noncompliance with treatment, that is, not taking the medications prescribed or taking them in dosages different from those prescribed. There are many reasons for noncompliance, ranging from the older individual's deficits in memory and comprehension to being unable to afford medications or treatments. The unpleasant side effects of medications, such as severe constipation, urinary retention, dizziness, sleepiness, blurred vision, and incoordination, are major factors in noncompliance. Even when the elderly use their medications properly, many commonly suffer from the negative consequences of using multiple drugs. These may include the unpleasant and sometimes harmful effects of drug interactions. Also, taking several drugs may exacerbate certain undesirable medication effects or lessen desirable ones.

It is especially important for psychiatrists and other mental-health workers to be knowledgeable about the metabolism and excretion of various medications in the aging; as people's bodies age, their responses to drugs change. For instance, older individuals usually suffer from diminished intestinal absorption of drugs. Decreased metabolism or enzymatic breakdown of drugs by the liver occurs, as well as decreased protein binding and less efficient kidney clearance. Consequently, it is highly likely that the ordinary dosage ranges of most of the available psychotropic (mind-affecting) medications must be reduced.

Present and Future Directions

Research

There are extensive research needs pertaining to almost every aspect of aging.

One of the most pressing needs is for epidemiological and demographic studies on elderly individuals with mental or psychiatric problems. Geographic variations in the prevalence of different types of disorders, this health-care-utilization practices of the elderly, the availability of services, and a variety of other matters need to be determined. A better actuarial and statistical base is a prerequisite for many research and policy matters pertaining to the mental health care of the elderly.

A muliplicity of factors affecting mental health need to be studied in more depth. They include the influence of sex differences and of the different ways and degrees in which people are vulnerable to psychiatric disorders. The relative age of onset of mental problems, familial and genetic tendencies, and predisposing and environmental factors also require elaboration.

For diagnostic purposes, it is essential to explore methods of early detection of mental illness. More precise classification systems of disease need to be developed, as well as methods of determining the ways in which cognitive deficits, affective (or emotional) disorders, and other forms of psychopathology may interact and complicate their diagnosis in the elderly. Classification systems should require clearer criteria for distinguishing dementia, delirium, and depression. Such systems should also specify the unique features of the various mental disorders of the elderly, including affective disorders, anxiety, psychotic disorders, psychosexual disorders, psychosomatic disorders, alcohol and drug abuse, and sleep and daily rhythm disturbances.

Basic research in the areas of neurochemistry, biochemistry, and physiology of the nervous system is required to clarify the nature of basic cellular dysfunctions and the dysfunctions of neurotransmitters (substances that transmit nerve impulses). These abnormal functionings underlie memory deficits, sleep disturbances, loss of vitality, pain, depression, sexual dysfunctions, and other forms of mental illness. The better we understand the causal mechanisms of these conditions, the greater the likelihood that we can develop more effective treatment.

Another important area for research about which little information is available is the identification of risk factors in the elderly that predict the likelihood of dementia, depression, suicide, psychosis, anxiety, and a variety of other common problems. Studies are also required to differentiate those changes associated with normal, healthy old age from those indicative of pathology. Such information is vital for determining the expected rate of various disorders and for policy decisions.

Along with these new sources of knowledge, efforts need to proceed in the further development of new technologies that will allow more in-depth investigations of brain function. Although nuclear magnetic-resonance imaging, computer axial tomography, cerebral-blood-flow analysis, and other diagnostic procedures have advanced our understanding of cerebral pathology, more sophisticated approaches are necessary for further breakthroughs.

Treatment

The treatment of the elderly presents a particular challenge to mental health workers largely, because it must be comprehensive and interdisciplinary. Treatment goals not only should pertain to the relief of pain and distress but should also aim to improve the quality of life and ensure optimal functioning.

More psychological services need to be available for both individual and group psychotherapy. This increase in availability will allow needy individuals to gain a better understanding of their problems and the reality of their situation and will also provide them with ways to improve their memory and functioning. Although elderly individuals are likely to be experiencing many deficits, the treatment emphasis needs to go beyond just coping with pain and disability. The strengths add future potential of individuals also need to be explored and enhanced.

Because pharmacological treatment constitutes a major part of any therapeutic approach for the elderly, the prescription of appropriate medications and the monitoring of their effects and the patient's treatment compliance require special attention. It is imperative that more effective drugs be developed to improve and preserve memory, to reduce further cognitive impairment, to alleviate depression with a minimum of adverse side effects, to diminish anxiety without risk of drug dependence and sedation, and to relieve chronic pain without the potential for drug addiction.

More effective drugs with fewer side effects would probably lead to less medication noncompliance. By taking the appropriate medications, elderly individuals presumably would have a better opportunity to benefit from treatment. For this to happen, mental health workers will need to establish better monitoring systems and to maintain greater awareness of the factors that diminish treatment compliance.

The comprehensive treatment of geriatric patients goes far beyond individual and group therapy and conferences with family guardians and other care workers. The mental health of the elderly is also very much dependent on many interactive services and agencies that address their physical, social, educational, and recreational needs.

Restorative and rehabilitative services, such as physical therapy and occupational therapy, are very important to the mental as well as the physical well-being of the elderly. Many other supportive services enhance the quality of life and thus the mental health of the elderly. Such services range from visiting nurses, homemakers or health aides, and meals on wheels, to financial counselors and escorts and telephone contacts. Participation in community agencies, such as senior citizens' groups, volunteer programs, and consumer councils, is very therapeutic for the elderly. The Elderhostel and other educational programs for the elderly have met an important intellectual need. Protective services and assistance with housing and shopping opportunities are also part of the comprehensive treatment of the elderly.

The home or a homelike residential facility seems to be a treatment setting superior to institutional or custodial care. To make such care possible, it is necessary to develop and provide a whole range of services and skilled personnel to work in such a context. Of necessity, this approach will require both family and community support.

From the above, it is apparent that an integrative, interdisciplinary approach is vital in providing optimal mental health care to elderly patients. This is dramatically illustrated in the treatment of Alzheimer's disease patients, who may or may not experience significant behavioral and emotional dysfunctions, and, in the treatment of depressed individuals. For such patients, family counseling and community liaisons are essential, and adequate psychiatric care must also usually involve neurological and medical consultation. Greater teamwork is desirable not only between psychiatrists and other physicians, but with social workers, psychologists, nurses, dentists, and podiatrists as well.

Legal Issues

With a rapidly expanding geriatric population, psychiatry will find itself increasingly involved in a variety of knotty legal issues, which, for resolution, will require close collaboration among other specialists as well as members of the judicial system. For instance, better and more precise criteria will need to be developed to define mental competency, especially for individuals whose cognitive abilities are primarily impaired or fluctuate in severity as a function of delirium, depression, agitation, or psychosis. The judgment regarding competence will determine if a legal guardian or conservator will be assigned to the individual. These agents not only are obligated to look after the affairs of their charges but may also become involved in institutional commitment or involuntary treatment proceedings.

The issue of mental competency, whether affected by organic or by psychiatric factors, has profound ramifications in the medical and mental health fields. The choice of who makes important decisions concerning the right to die and the consent to or refusal of surgery or medication or other treatment hinges on the judgment of competence. Whether a person is deemed mentally competent or not is a major factor in decisions concerning the validity of wills and bequests.

In order to safeguard the rights of elderly individuals, it is apparent that psychiatry and the legal system will need to work closely together to develop more precise and objective criteria for mental competency so that unnecessary conflict and expense will be reduced.

Prevention and Education

The major thrust of any national program concerned with the mental health needs of the elderly should be prevention. A number of steps can be taken to decrease the prospects of disease and to improve the situation of the aging in the long run.

For example, it may well be the case that much of the depression associated with aging will be diminished if individuals are better prepared earlier in their lives for the problems likely to lie ahead. Such preparation may involve the initiation of educational programs in the workplace many years before retirement that will encourage and enable individuals to develop alternative interests or to learn how to appreciate not having to work. Also, a new educational curriculum may need to be developed that teaches people about the entire life cycle and that attempts to train them to use suitable coping techniques for the problems they may encounter as they age. This curriculum could be introduced in high school and college, in industry, or in the community.

Also, in the area of prevention, instituting certain lifestyle changes may ensure a fuller and happier life and thereby diminish the prospects of such debilitating symptoms as depression, fatigue, and insomnia. These lifestyle changes include proper nutrition, exercise programs, relaxation techniques, socialization, and community involvement all of which promote a feeling of well-being.

At a broader level, the public needs to become better educated about the growing mental-health-care requirements of the elderly. This education can be done through the government's sponsorship of various community education programs, and efforts need to be made as well to exploit the mass communication media. A better educated public can make more enlightened decisions about establishing social priorities.

Training

Because of the growing mental-health needs of the elderly, a more concerted effort must be made to recruit competent individuals to work in the field. By its very nature, geriatric psychiatry requires an extremely broad base of knowledge, not only psychiatry, medicine, and neurology, but also in the principles of psychology, sociology, and economics. Because such broadly based knowledge is unlikely to be available to casual or inexperienced workers in psychiatry, it is becoming increasingly important that responsible and concerned health planners make certain that future physicians and psychiatrists are competent in the management and treatment of elderly individuals.

Part of the answer is to provide medical students with more instruction in geriatric psychiatry.

Part of the answer is to expose psychiatric residents to more elderly patients and to train them to become more knowledgeable about the special problems and requirements of the elderly.

And part of the answer is to further encourage the development of the subspecialty of geriatric psychiatry by establishing approved training programs and appropriate specialty boards to certify individuals as having mastered the requisite body of knowledge in this complex area. To accomplish this goal, it may be necessary to increase the number of training centers where interested physicians can obtain fellowship training in geriatric psychiatry or can participate in appropriate postdoctoral programs. As part of their training experience, qualified individuals should be required to work closely with all appropriate medical and nonmedical professionals involved in the care of the elderly. They will also need to become knowledgeable about the wide spectrum of community services and facilities available to aging persons.

Social Policy

Any effective medical-psychiatric approach to the elderly will require major changes in social policy. Medicare coverage for psychiatric outpatient services is inadequate; it provides fewer benefits for psychiatric care than for other medical treatments. Any governmental policy that appears to regard mental problems as less significant than medical problems must be corrected.

Another major social policy will require a decision about the main locus of care for elderly individuals. If it is determined that home care rather than institutional care is the most humane and beneficial approach, then there will be profound implications for programmatic practices and the allocation of personnel and other resources. Home care, for example, will require visitations by mental health workers, scheduled activities within the home, and the availability of transportation if office visits or special diagnostic evaluations are needed.

With the proliferation of the various local, state, and national governmental agencies concerned with the issues of aging, it is increasingly important for these groups to coordinate their efforts better to realize their aims. Better coordination will result in an increase in the resources and money that can be used to address all the issues affecting the aging.

Summary and Recommendations

In summary, then, funding will be required for basic and clinical research programs covering every aspect of aging.

Treatment programs for the elderly will require the establishment of a broader range of services and of mechanisms for matching patient needs with resources. A continuum of care would go as follows: private outpatient therapy, visits to community mental-health clinics, nursing-home visits by psychiatric professionals, short-term residential treatment, day care, foster home care, private psychiatric hospitalization, and prolonged institutional care. Community-based services could include home visits, recreational therapy, community service centers, and vocational rehabilitation.

In the legal area, psychiatrists and mental health personnel will need to work much more closely with patient representatives and guardians in determining the best interests of their patients and in safeguarding their individual rights.

The public will need to become better educated about the special needs of the elderly and about how later problems may be avoided.

In order to increase the numbers of qualified professionals working in geriatric mental health, major shifts in medical and psychiatric training will have to take place. New models of mental health care must be developed that are not only therapeutically efficient and cost-effective but also interdisciplinary and integrative. These new models may also involve the use of novel housing arrangements, such as group homes, shared living, or other, more appropriate settings that will become an important component of therapy.

To accomplish these goals, a major social commitment is necessary. This commitment will require increased funding and resources.

Selected Bibliography

Anderson, J. M., and Cartwright, W. S., The National Institute of Aging's health care expenditure model. In G. L. Maddox and E. W. Busse (eds.), *Aging: The Universal Human Experience*. New York: Springer, 1987.

Blazer, D. G., The epidemiology of psychiatric disorders in late life. In E. W. Busse and D. G. Blazer, *Geriatric Psychiatry*. Washington, DC: American Psychiatric Press, 1989.

Bluestone, H., Travin, S., and Kaufman, M., Administrative and forensic considerations in the operation of a geriatric psychiatry service. In R. Rosner and H. I. Schwartz (eds.), *Geriatric Psychiatry and the Law* (pp. 205–240). New York: Plenum, 1987.

Busse, E. W., and Blazer, D. G., The future of geriatric psychiatry. In E. W. Busse and D. G. Blazer, *Geriatric Psychiatry*. Washington, DC: American Psychiatric Press, 1989.

Butler, R. N., and Leurs, M. I., *Aging and Mental Health*. St. Louis, MO: C. V. Mosby, 1982.

Charatan, F. B., Geriatric psychiatry: Legal and forensic issues. In R.

Rosner and H. I. Schwartz (eds.), *Geriatric Psychiatry and the Law* (pp. 3–16). New York: Plenum, 1987.

Cristofolo, V. J., and Hayflick, L., Basic biological research in aging: An overview. In G. L. Maddox and E. W. Busse (eds.), *Aging: The Universal Human Experience*. New York: Springer, 1987.

Crooks, V., Impact of social policy and planning issues on geriatric mental health care. In J. P. Abrahaus and V. Crooks (eds.), *Geriatric Mental Health*. Orlando, FL: Greene and Stratton, 1984.

Eisdorfer, C., Models of mental health care of the elderly. In J. P. Abrahaus and V. Crooks (eds.), *Geriatric Mental Health*. Orlando, FL: Greene and Stratton, 1984.

Kramer, M., Taube, C. A., and Redick, R. W., Patterns of use of psychiatric facilities by the ages: Past, present, and future. In C. Eisdorfer and M. P. Lawton (eds.), *The Psychology of Adult Development and Aging*. Washington, DC: American Psychological Association, 1973.

Maddox, G. L., and Glass, T. A., The continuum of care: Movement toward the community. In E. W. Busse and D. G. Blazer, *Geriatric Psychiatry*. Washington, DC: American Psychiatric Press, 1989.

Promoting Health/Preventing Disease: Objectives for the Nation, USDHSS, Public Health Service, Government Printing Office, Washington, DC, 1980.

Salzman, C., *Clinical Geriatric Psychopharmacology*. New York: McGraw-Hill, 1984.

Silverstone, B. M., Beyond the one to one treatment relationship. In L. Bellak and T. B. Karasu, *Geriatric Psychiatry*. New York: Greene and Stratton, 1976.

Straus, R., Alcohol problems among the elderly: The need for a biobehavioral perspective. In George Maddox, Lee N. Robins, and Nathan Rosenberg (eds.), *Nature and Extent of Alcohol Problems among the Elderly* (pp. 9–28). Research Monograph No. 14, National Institute on Alcohol Abuse and Alcoholism, Rockville, Maryland, 1984.

Straus, R., Risk factors in geriatric drug use: Biobehavioral issues. In Steven R. Moore and Thomas W. Teal (eds.), *Geriatric Drug Use: Clinical and Social Perspectives* (pp. 160–167). New York: Pergamon Press, 1985.

Taylor, R. C., Current developments in identifying the elderly at risk. In G. L. Maddox and E. W. Busse (eds.), *Aging: The Universal Human Experience*. New York: Springer, 1987.

13

The Benefits of Psychotherapy for the Elderly

ARNOLD M. LEVIN, PH.D., B.C.D., L.C.S.W.

Introduction

This presentation describes some of the ways in which clinical social workers use psychodynamic psychotherapy to help the elderly. Until recently, many psychotherapists considered the elderly too rigid to benefit from therapy, and many of the elderly and their families agreed. More and more, those of us who work with the elderly are learning that they use psychotherapy effectively. They can change their ways of thinking about life, increase their feelings of well-being, decrease their feelings of depression, improve their relationships with significant others, and increase their life satisfaction. In other words, we have come to recognize that life can change and people can grow at any time during the cycle of life.

Appropriate Therapy

Many different theories guide psychotherapy, including many different psychodynamic theories. The essential thrust of psychodynamic therapy is to help a person come to understand the meaning of his or her behavior and feelings. This approach differs from cognitive therapy somewhat, and it differs considerably from the behavior-modification and pharmacological approaches. The premise of the psychodynamic approach is that the more you understand the meaning of your feelings, behavior, and reactions, the more likely you are to be the master of your life and behavior, to be the driver rather than to be driven by poorly understood, even mysterious, urges.

Competent, well-educated therapists choose the therapy that seems most appropriate to the client. In no way does this imply an opportunistic approach. Rather, it is suggested as an antidote to the sad reality that therapists too often attempt to fit the client to the theory rather than the theory to the client. The most appropriate stance for the therapist is to regard the client as the expert about herself or himself, and the therapist's main responsibility is to help the client achieve even greater expertise. The therapist learns from the client with the client's assistance, by listening carefully and understanding intellectually and emotionally.

Transference and Countertransference

This business of listening and understanding is, of course, at the heart of all human relationships, including those between client and therapist. Therapists use two special concepts to help them listen more meaningfully and with deeper understanding than most of us do in everyday interactions. These concepts are transference and countertransference.

Transference refers to the ubiquitous human propensity to bring to today's relationships or situations emotionally powerful meanings that are carried over from past experiences. These meanings are usually "transferred" outside the person's consciousness, or unconsciously. For example, I am reminded of an elderly woman whose mother had often been late, and sometimes forgetful, about calling for her at school and other activities. In her mind, this woman equated her mother's forgetfulness with lack of love and even created a "love thermometer" to measure degrees of lovingness based on mothers' timeliness in picking up their children. She had completely "forgotten" this childhood experience. Recently, however, she had been waiting for her own children to pick her up for an important family event. They were significantly delayed by traffic. She reacted with an explosive rage way beyond the momentary irritation, much to her own consternation as well as that of her children. In therapy, she came to understand that she had transferred her early-childhood rage to the current situation. She was relieved in recognizing that she had not become an "old witch." And she was able to apologize and mend fences with her children, especially with her daughter-in-law; everyone felt better. Unfortunately, insights into transference reactions are not easily come by. Fortunately, a psychotherapist who listens carefully may often catalyze the process.

Countertransference is the term that therapists use to refer to their own reactions that get in the way of helping people whom they have set out to help. For example, a therapist sought my consultation regarding a sixtyish man who had looked to him for help in resolving a serious marital disruption, with the possibility of divorce. The therapist prematurely jumped to reassure his client that, at this middle-aged time of his life, he might feel better off "going it alone." To this, the client responded forcefully that (he didn't want to divorce;) he longed for an intimate relationship with his wife and wanted to focus on how to attain it. The young unmarried therapist came to realize that his empathic failure to understand his client was related to unconscious feelings of his own that stemmed from his life experience. He was personally in conflict about committing himself to an ongoing intimate relationship.

Complexity of the Elderly

In many ways, the treatment of the elderly differs little from the treatment of younger clients. In other ways, it differs considerably. It needs always to be kept in mind that "the elderly" do not constitute a homogeneous group of people who may be lumped together into a special psychological category.

Studies indicate that elderly people tend to be more highly differentiated from each other, more complex, than are younger people. There are many reasons, not the least of which is the unpredictability of the physical, psychological, economic, and social situation of the individual older person. In addition, the elderly inevitably have an increasing variation in their historical experience with increasing years, including intense involvement for longer time spans with many more people.

Interestingly, recent research suggests that one of the strongest predictors of good life satisfaction among people over sixty-five is the existence of a close relationship from early childhood on with one or more siblings. Too often, sibling relationships have been ignored by therapists and others.

Therapists' Feelings toward the Elderly

Therapists' feelings toward the elderly also tend to be more complicated. For example, a therapist in her forties, when confronted with a client in her eighties, had great difficulty in accepting the all-too-obvious fact that the elderly woman was suffering from serious depression. The therapist attempted to minimize the problems, which prevented work toward their resolution. In consultation, the therapist revealed her fears of her own aging and the inevitability of her own death, hoped that all her own problems would disappear as she grew older, and feared her own aging parents' problems, including their transitory depression and the inevitability of their death. Discussion freed the therapist to listen more empathically to and in greater attunement with her elderly client.

In another instance, a nurse was confronted by an elderly patient who was in mourning over a recent loss, had begun losing weight rapidly, and was giving away her possessions as though preparing to die. The nurse's personal and professional sensibilities were seriously upset because she saw it as her responsibility to preserve the patient's life at all costs. In consultation, it was revealed that the nurse's own parents had been killed in an accident that she had always felt she should have prevented.

As the nurse felt more comfortable, she was able to talk with her elderly patient more freely and acceptingly rather than judgmentally about the patient's ambivalence toward living or dying. That is, the nurse was able to relate to her patient without her own internal filters preventing "listening and understanding." She no longer had to "rescue" the patient, as she had been unable rescue her own parents. With the therapist's acceptance of the patient, the patient's depression lifted enough to curtail her weight loss, and the nurse felt more competent about doing her job. She had made herself available to learning from the patient. And the patient had profited.

An Ornery Patient

Although clinicians practice psychotherapy primarily in their consulting rooms, it is not an exotic, mysterious process. Therapeutic interventions may take place anywhere, including in hospitals, in nursing homes, in centers where seniors gather for various purposes, or in their own homes.

I offer a vignette here of an intervention by an internist in a hospital that represents a "psychotherapeutic" intervention, although there was no explicit agreement to do psychotherapy. The situation was the following.

A woman in her eighties had been hospitalized for the treatment of several serious, life-threatening physical conditions. She stirred up great anger among the hospital staff because of her "refusal to cooperate," her "orneriness," her refusal to respond to English-speaking people, and her other "obnoxious behavior." The internist, who was especially sensitive, concerned, and creative, asked the patient's daughter to tell him about her mother. It turned out that she was an Armenian woman who had survived pogroms carried out by Turkish people early in this century. She had established a newspaper to tell her people's story to the world. She had corresponded privately with leaders of great nations.

Altogether, this "ornery patient" turned out to be a rather remarkable person. The wise internist persuaded his patient to tell him her story. He communicated what he had learned to the hospital staff. They began treating the patient more sympathetically. Lo and behold, the "ornery patient" responded by becoming charmingly cooperative in working in her own behalf—in English.

An Instructive Example

Encapsulated in this vignette are many elements illustrative of the plight of the elderly when confronted with illness, as well as some of the difficulties encountered by caregivers. It is an instructive example. Here we have an elderly woman who had been relatively independent, a leader, and a fighter for a righteous cause. She had used her talents actively for her own survival and that of others. Her self-esteem had been built on that personality stance. She was one of those "tough old birds" who had suffered through the vicissitudes of life and prevailed. She was a survivor. She had been a competent person all her life. Until now. Illness had laid her low. She had been rendered helpless and dependent on others. She had to suffer intrusive procedures to cure or ameliorate her illness. The major psychological techniques and internal resources on which she had depended throughout her life to maintain her self-esteem had been rendered inoperative. Yet, she had to cope somehow.

What she did to cope was to regress to earlier infantile ways of coping, namely, to rebel in an infantile way against what she perceived as assaults by her helpers. To be "ornery" was to hold onto some semblance of power. To her caretakers, what was visible was irritating, unacceptable behavior. The concept of "empowering" the elderly is easier for helping professionals to pay lip service to than to act on. As the patient's behavior became more regressive and as she resisted efforts to help her, she frustrated the helpers' mission to help. They felt helpless and reacted with anger. To reach an understanding of the meaning of the patient's behavior and of their own reactions to it, the helpers had to stretch beyond the overt manifestations. When the internist found a way to get his patient to tell her story, he tapped into the essence of all psychotherapies. To tell one's story, to have it heard, understood, accepted, and even admired, is central to psychotherapy. Older people, like younger ones, want and need to be heard.

In this example, a relatively quick psychological "cure" was effected through a simple intervention. The physician used his intuitive empathy to talk with the patient. The patient was enabled to recover symbolically, through reminiscence, some of her earlier life techniques for maintaining her self-esteem and feelings of competence. As a result, she was able to relinquish regressive infantile ways of coping with feelings of helplessness. Nowhere in this instance did anyone think about transference or countertransference. No one regarded what he or she was doing as psychotherapy; the goals of intervention were pragmatic and immediate. Yet, from my view as a clinical social worker, many of the elements of ordinary psychotherapy operated in this case. The greater part of the educational preparation of psychotherapists is devoted to understanding these concepts and bringing them to life. Not everyone is as intuitively gifted and committed as the internist I have used here illustratively.

Therapists do not change, cure, or rescue people. Each of us is responsible for her or his own growth, change, and mastery. The therapist is a catalytic enabler. Because one of the most frequently encountered desires among the elderly is to make sense of their lives, to find the meaning in it, psychodynamic therapy, with its emphasis on understanding the meanings of feelings, behavior, and reactions, seems especially appropriate for them. Older people want and need to tell their story. Therapy, in its essence, entails people's telling their tales so that they can be understood and so that they may understand themselves.

The Jealous Grandmother

I present another poignant example that more nearly conforms to ordinary psychotherapy. This vignette illustrates that the elderly come to elderliness with all their personality idiosyncrasies, their special histories, their special ways of defending themselves against hurts, their special ways of maintaining their self-esteem and feelings of competence, their special fears, and sometimes their special undiagnosed defects, which have dogged them in unrecognized ways all their lives.

A clinical social worker saw a sixty-five-year-old woman who was depressed. Eventually, the woman confessed that she was deeply ashamed of herself because she was so jealous of her three-year-old granddaughter. She was jealous of the ease with which the little girl could communicate with her mother and with her baby sister, verbally and through physical communication, a kind of mutually empathic communication. It turned out that this grandmother had always had difficulty expressing herself verbally or in writing. Her own mother had always considered her either dumb or recalcitrant and stubbornly resistant. The clinical social worker, who had experience with children with learning defects, began to suspect that grandmother may have been an undiagnosed learning-disabled child. She discussed this possibility, the grandmother agreed to undergo an evaluation, and they found that she did indeed suffer from a severe learning disability.

The grandmother experienced a profound sense of relief in discovering, after all those sixty-five years, that she did have a disability, that it was identifiable, nameable, and understandable, and that it was not a global deficiency. Her envy of her children and grandchildren could now be understood as reality-based. Because she now felt for the first time that she had been understood, and her pain had been acknowledged by another, her therapist, her shame was dissipated, her depression lifted, and she could finally function wholeheartedly as the grandmother she was and wanted to be.

This example illustrates the principle that, in work with the elderly, it is of vital importance to call on all the knowledge that we have collectively, as professionals, not only about the elderly, but about humans throughout the life cycle.

Special Stresses of the Elderly, and Their Families and Caregivers

Special stresses are likely to afflict the elderly, their caring families, their caretakers, and the professional helpers who work with them. Following is a list of those stresses.

The stresses of old age include:

- Unresolved conflicts from earlier life.
- Undiagnosed defects that may have gone unacknowledged throughout the lifetime and that may become especially painful in later life.
- Interpersonal losses.
- Physical disabilities.
- Loss of external manifestations of the self.
- Loss of roles.
- Loss of defensive outlets.
- Forced reliance on caretakers.
- Confrontations with death.
- Conflict over the wish to live versus the wish to die.

In addition to all of these, there may be special insults that the elderly have not resolved. For instance, a recently widowed seventy-year-old woman who had discovered in her lost spouse's effects evidence of earlier affairs was confronted with questions about the meaningfulness of her life and about its integrity. She had feelings of betrayal and wondered about her own "foolishness" in having been "taken in." Feelings like these need to be responded to, and the person needs to be helped to come to terms with herself and with the lost mate as part of making of her life a meaningful whole.

The stresses of family members who are caretakers include:

- Fear of loss and becoming orphaned.
- Fear of repeating ancient childhood narcissistic insults.

- Guilt over not being adequate caretakers.
- Ambivalence.
- Competitiveness with siblings.
- Fears about rage.
- Fears about their own vulnerability and mortality and about being "next."

Many of these fears are similar to those experienced by younger professionals called on to work with the elderly. It is of the greatest importance that professional helpers—whether they be clinical social workers or members of the other helping professions—be aware that these kinds of feelings may influence their work with the elderly. The feelings are not "bad." They are just there, and we need to be alert to their presence to guard against their limiting our usefulness.

Summary

This chapter describes a psychodynamically oriented clinical-social-work view of work with the elderly. It emphasizes that psychotherapy may be very useful to the elderly. It suggests that struggle, change, growth, and development may occur at any point in the life cycle. It also suggests that, although there are various theories of psychotherapy, the wise therapist tailors the theory to the client, not the client to the theory. The chapter defines some of the special ways clinicians listen, attempt to be attuned to the client, and understand. It takes the mystery out of some basic theoretical concepts like transference and countertransference while explaining their importance as therapeutic tools. It reminds us that the elderly are not a simple, homogeneous group but are, in fact, even more differentiated than other age groups. It argues that therapists who work with the elderly need to be alert to all aspects of knowledge about how humans develop throughout the life cycle, including early childhood, taking into account all the special problems and stresses that may arise at different points in the life cycle and their manifestations in the later years.

14

Neurology of Aging

The Problem of Dementia in the Year 2000

RICHARD MAYEUX, M.D.

Summary

With advancing age, nearly every person experiences a chronic disabling illness, and dementia is one of the more common disabling conditions of the elderly. The demented patient requires both extended health care services and assistance with activities of daily life, such as eating, dressing, and bathing. The frequency of dementia increases significantly with age, so that by age eighty-five as many as the 45 percent of elderly people could be considered demented. Because our society is currently aging at an extremely rapid pace, it is likely that an "epidemic" of dementia will be faced as early as the "baby-boom" generation reaches retirement age.

The causes of dementia are variable, but by far the most common cause is Alzheimer's disease. This is followed by dementia with stroke (either as the result of the stroke or in conjunction with another condition) and dementia with Parkinson's disease. Together, these three disorders account for 80 percent of the cases of dementia in older adults.

The frequency of Alzheimer's disease rises steadily after age sixty-five. At sixty-five, the prevalence of the condition in the population at large is about 10 percent, but it is nearly four times this at age eighty-five. The incidence, or number of new cases developing over time, also increases very rapidly. There is no known risk factor for Alzheimer's disease except advanced age and heredity. Several epidemiological studies point to a high familial occurrence of Alzheimer's disease, and laboratory studies now link the young-onset form to a specific chromosome (chromosome 21). It is clear, however, that not all types of Alzheimer's disease are linked to this chromosome. Therefore, the search for other clues to the etiology of Alzheimer's disease continues.

Parkinson's disease, like Alzheimer's disease, is a disorder of the aging nervous system. Both the prevalence and the incidence double with each decade of life after age sixty-five. Although typically regarded as a disorder of motility, or movement, between 10 and 30 percent of patients with Parkinson's disease become demented. In particular, the patient who develops the motor manifestations after age seventy has a four times greater likelihood of also becoming demented. Because dementia limits the use of the conventional treatment of Parkinson's disease, mortality may increase in these patients. The pathology of dementia in patients with Parkinson's disease shares many of the morphological, or structural, and biochemical features of Alzheimer's disease, suggesting a more than coincidental link. As with Alzheimer's disease, the only known risk factors of dementia in patients with Parkinson's disease are advanced age and a family history of dementia.

In general, stroke is more common than either Alzheimer's disease or Parkinson's disease, but dementia is not a constant feature of stroke. Nevertheless, stroke-related dementia, or so-called multi-infarct dementia, is the second leading cause of dementia in the elderly after Alzheimer's disease. There is no consistent pattern or disease process that accounts for this high frequency. Many stroke patients also have Alzheimer's disease, but many do not, a finding that suggests that the underlying vascular disease may play an etiological, or causal, role. Hypertension, the volume of the brain affected by the stroke, and the stroke's location may all be causal factors. The prevalence and incidence of stroke dementia also increase rapidly with advanced age. There are no known risk factors for stroke-related dementia. Multiple strokes, particularly those in the posterior cerebral artery, are most often encountered.

Lewis Thomas, oncologist, essayist, and author of *Lives of a Cell,* may be correct in stating that Alzheimer's disease is the "disease of the century." His statement may need to be extended as an even greater number of our elderly become demented in the next century.

Introduction

In 1987, the National Institute on Aging (NIA) reported to Congress that the elderly population over age sixty-five had been increasing at the rate of 2 percent annually, or about 750,000 persons per year, since 1985. The report predicted that this pace would continue until the year 2020. The greatest increase would occur after the year 2000, when the baby-boom generation enters the elderly category.

People over age eighty-five are the most rapidly growing segment of our society, increasing at a rate of 4 percent per year, whereas the segment under sixty-five increases at about 1 percent annually. In 1987, there were twenty-three million people over age sixty-five in the United States, but by 2020, there will be that many individuals over age seventy-five.

The report by the NIA also noted that most older adults develop one or more chronic health problems. Chronic illness will, no doubt, continue to be the most important cause of disability in this age group, although the degree of dependence on others that is associated with the disability varies from minimal to complete, depending on the type of illness. In 1984, it was estimated that three million people over the age of sixty-five were disabled enough to require some help with activities of daily living. Another million required even more help with routine daily activities such as bathing, dressing, and eating. Disability caused by diseases of the nervous system will surely require increasing amounts of care and professional health services. Diseases causing loss of mental function (dementia), paralysis, and loss of mobility rapidly escalate the cost of caring for the disabled elderly person.

Dementia, in terms of functional disability in the elderly, may be the most debilitating condition. Alzheimer's disease alone accounts for over 70 percent of the causes of dementia among the aged. In private practice, a neurologist can expect to see 1 patient with dementia for every 2 patients with stroke, or stated in different terms, almost 2 out of every 100 patients seen in neurological consultation are likely to be demented.

Dementia has become a major health problem only in the past few decades. Improved sanitation, public immunization, and antibiotics have decreased the threat of infection, thereby increasing life expectancy and postponing death. Because the rates of dementia increase rapidly with advanced age, and because mortality has also declined with improved medical care, dementia can only increase as the population of the United States ages.

Epidemiological studies (epidemiology is the science that studies the incidence, distribution, and control of disease in populations) provide vital information concerning the number of new cases to be expected in the future. Moreover, current population studies indicate a dramatic increase in the number of elderly who are at greatest risk for dementia. Some physicians have considered dementia a syndrome that includes general categories of neuropsychiatric disorders, such as organic brain syndrome or senile psychosis. Investigations have used more refined, criteria-based diagnoses and have attempted to be disease-specific. Standard measures of duration and severity still vary depending on the underlying disorder, however.

This review focuses on what is likely to be the impending epidemic of dementia, called the neurological burden for the twenty-first century. I attempt to include the available information on the frequency and distribution of dementia. *Frequency* refers to how often dementia occurs in the population, and *distribution* refers to which segment(s) of the population gets a disease and in what proportion. I also discuss the risk factors for the most common causes of dementia, and I am disease-specific where possible but remain within the limitations of diagnostic accuracy for certain disorders.

Epidemiology of Dementia

The prevalence, or the proportion in any given population, of severe dementia, of any type, is currently estimated to be between 1.3 to 6.2 percent of people over age sixty-five. If milder degrees of intellectual impairment are included, the estimates are even higher, from 2.6 to 15.4 percent. A recent study found the prevalence of dementia in residents of an East Boston community to rise dramatically after age eighty-five, to 45 percent, nearly double what had been found in previous studies. It was concluded that a greater number of elderly individuals than previously acknowledged were becoming disabled by dementia in late life.

The incidence of dementia, or the number of new cases developing in a population over time, has been difficult to ascertain retrospectively, but rates between 1.4 and 2.3 percent annually have been found. One study showed incidence rates of .43 percent for ages sixty to sixty-four and 3.3 percent after age eighty. In that study, the risk or probability of developing Alzheimer's disease was as high as 27 percent by age sixty and continued to climb to 31 percent by age ninety. Similar rates have been found in other studies.

Alzheimer's Disease

By far, the most common form of dementia is Alzheimer's disease, but the cause is unknown. The diagnosis is based on both clinical evidence of intellectual impairment during life and pathological evidence at an autopsy of a characteristic morphological, or structural, triad. Researchers have considered genetic, toxic, immunological, metabolic, and traumatic risk factors in Alzheimer's disease, but all are unproven. The only known risk factor for sporadic Alzheimer's disease is advanced age; the incidence and prevalence increase dramatically with each decade of life after age sixty. The accuracy of clinical diagnosis in living patients is, at best, 82 to 90 percent. Investigations of Alzheimer's disease have differed in diagnostic criteria, methods of ascertaining cases, and age distribution. Parkinson's disease and stroke, other common nervous-system disorders of the elderly, may also occur in conjunction with Alzheimer's disease. But individuals with these diseases, because of their other diagnoses, are likely to have been excluded, and therefore underestimated, in epidemiological investigations of Alzheimer's disease.

The prevalence of clinically diagnosed Alzheimer's disease was recently reviewed. For people sixty-five and older, the prevalence ranged from .39 percent in Turku, Finland, to 5.8 percent in Great Britain. This wide variation in rates probably reflects differences in diagnostic criteria and case ascertainment as discussed above. Even with the wide variation, it is clear that the prevalence of clinically diagnosed Alzheimer's disease increases with each decade. In nearly all the studies, the prevalence rate more than doubles between the sixtieth and eightieth years of life.

The increase in the population over age sixty-five in developed countries over the next several years will be accompanied by a dramatic increase in the proportion of the population suffering from Alzheimer's disease. In France, for example, a 9 percent increase in prevalence is expected by the year 2000, and in Japan, a 76.6 percent increase is projected. The United States falls in the middle, at 42 percent by that time.

The incidence rate of clinically diagnosed Alzheimer's disease also rises acutely with advanced age. For all people over sixty, the rates of individuals diagnosed with new cases of Alzheimer's disease each year has varied from a low estimate of .069 percent in Finland to .12 percent in Sweden. The differences in rates have been attributed to whether or not other diagnoses were included, such as senile psychosis and multi-infarct dementia, or stroke. A more recent investigation using strict diagnostic criteria for dementia found an incidence rate of .12 to .20 percent annually in Rochester, Minnesota, for people over thirty years of age. Again, a steady increase was found in the age group over seventy-five.

Risk Factors

Disease correlates or risk factors for Alzheimer's disease have been difficult to investigate because of the potential for misclassification of patients as well as the difficulty in obtaining medical histories. The spouse or a child has most often been interviewed about potential exposures during the patient's lifetime. Most consider these data of limited value. Nonetheless, the most important risk factor identified has been a family history of dementia, particularly in a sibling.

Some research suggests that there may be a genetic cause for Alzheimer's disease. In one study, four independent families, each of which had one or more members with Alzheimer's disease, had the same chromosomal abnormality. Several case-control studies have provided evidence of prevalence in particular families supporting a genetic cause. Some investigators have reported that, among first-degree relatives (children, brothers, and sisters) of patients with Alzheimer's disease (regardless of the age of onset), as many as 50 percent will manifest an Alzheimer-like dementia by the eighth decade of life. However, others do not share this belief. A genetic cause for Alzheimer's disease remains a subject of controversy. Controversy also exists concerning the nature of the familial Alzheimer's disease gene, but this controversy should be resolved with further study. Although some risk factors seem more likely than others, none can yet be completely eliminated.

Parkinson's Disease

Parkinson's disease is a chronic progressive nerve disease, usually of later life, marked by a tremor and weakness of resting muscles and by a peculiar gait. The role of Parkinson's disease in the etiology, or development, of dementia is confusing. Although Parkinsonism is not typically considered a cause of dementia, patients with Parkinson's disease, in certain studies, have been found to have mental deterioration more frequently than do the healthy elderly. A recent incidence study indicated that dementia with Parkinson's disease may be the third most common manifestation of dementia overall. Autopsies show both neurological and biochemical evidence that point to the simultaneous occurrence of Parkinson's disease and Alzheimer's disease. Although not all demented patients with Parkinson's disease exhibit the pathological changes of Alzheimer's disease, this research implies that there may be more than a causal relationship between these two common diseases of the elderly.

The prevalence of Parkinson's disease ranges from about .1 to .2 percent overall, and there are no known sex, racial, or ethnic differences in those who develop the disease. However, over age sixty-five, there is a dramatic increase from .85 to 1.2 percent, and the prevalence twice that in all lower age ranges. The prevalence again doubles after age seventy-five.

The incidence of Parkinson's disease arising from unknown causes also rises dramatically with age. Some scientists have found the rate to be greater between the ages of sixty-five and seventy-four (.1 percent per year) and even greater at ages seventy-five to eighty-four (.25 percent per year).

There is some confusion and controversy about how many patients with Parkinson's disease also experience mental deterioration, or dementia. Differing criteria for diagnosing dementia, plus different research methods, probably account for the various results. Depending on the criteria used, between 11 and 29 percent of Parkinson's disease patients also have dementia. The prevalence of mental deterioration is 2 to $2\frac{1}{2}$ times higher for those over age seventy (between 25 and 33 percent) than for those under seventy (10.5 to 17.6 percent).

Preliminary studies suggest that people with Parkinson's disease have a higher probability of developing dementia than people who do not have Parkinson's. Also, as people age, the severity of their dementia increases.

Risk Factors for Dementia in Patients with Parkinson's Disease

The only known risk factor for dementia with Parkinson's disease is the onset of the motor manifestations at an advanced age. Some drugs used to treat Parkinson's disease may bring on acute confusion in Parkinsonian patients, even in nondemented patients with Parkinson's disease. Although demented patients more often develop problems on these drugs, researchers have found that some nondemented patients also became confused. Several scientists recently reported that demented patients with Parkinson's disease had a slightly greater number of demented relatives than did nondemented patients with Parkinson's disease.

Stroke

Stroke is the sudden lessening or loss of consciousness, sensation, and voluntary motion usually caused by cerebrovascular disease or atherosclerosis, both of which entail the rupture or obstruction of an artery to the brain. Although stroke is the second most common cause of dementia, the mechanism by which it causes dementia remains an enigma. Some of the same tissue changes of Alzheimer's disease are often present in demented patients with cerebrovascular disease. The particular area of injury produced by a stroke or a series of strokes may also result in a clinical syndrome resembling dementia. This syndrome has been termed *multi-infarct dementia,* suggesting an origin of disease that remains unproven. It is estimated that between 20 and 25 percent of all cases of dementia are due to stroke, and another 10 to 15 percent of patients have a combination of Alzheimer's disease and stroke. However, only a few epidemiological studies exist.

Prevalence studies of dementia in patients with stroke are few. In one study, 9 of 50 patients were considered demented as a result of cerebral softening due to stroke; 9 others had both Alzheimer's disease and stroke as the cause. In another study 72

(27.9 percent) of 258 demented patients were found to have dementia on the basis of stroke. In other studies, the prevalence has varied from 3.7 to 13.6 percent.

The results in the Stroke Data Bank of examinations of patients at four centers may yield better estimates than those in the literature. Although dementia was not formally assessed, the examining neurologists at each center judged whether or not the patient was demented. A probable cause (e.g., stroke-related, coincident with Alzheimer's disease, or other) was also recorded. Patients deemed untestable because of alterations in consciousness or severe aphasia were excluded.

Of the 1,267 patients from the four centers, 120 (12.1 percent) were considered demented (277 were untestable). At one center, the researchers suspected that, in 56.7 percent of the demented patients, coincidence with Alzheimer's disease was the cause of dementia, not the stroke. Although these data need more rigorous confirmation, they are particularly valuable because they are not based on a population preselected for dementia. More important, with neuropsychological testing to improve sensitivity, an even higher prevalence rate may be found.

There is even less information about the incidence of dementia following stroke. In one study, fifty-two patients under age sixty-five were followed after they had had a stroke. None of the patients had clinical or historical evidence of dementia before or three months after the stroke. However, during the four years of follow-up, three patients became demented according to the criteria used. No accompanying conditions were apparent; two of the patients had multiple strokes, and one had a single stroke. Three other patients began to show mental deterioration but did not reach the criteria for dementia by the end of the study.

After one year, the percentage of new cases of dementia in the New York Stroke Data Bank was approximately 6.0 percent. As with Alzheimer's disease and Parkinson's disease, the rates of new cases rose rapidly with each decade of life. Between the ages of sixty-five and sixty-nine, the rate was 6.5 percent, but between ages eighty and eighty-four, it was 15.8 percent. Again, these data need to be confirmed, but it is likely that stroke increases the risk of dementia in the elderly.

How stroke causes dementia is uncertain. At least six possible relationships between stroke and dementia have been suggested: a volume effect from a single large infarct, multiple infarcts, diffuse white-matter disease, posterior-cerebral-artery distribution strokes, border-zone or watershed infarcts, and, finally, coincidence with Alzheimer's disease.

Risk Factors for Dementia with Stroke

Because there are at least six mechanisms by which stroke and dementia are related, it is difficult to determine a single risk factor. There are likely to be several. It is possible that patients with stroke-related dementia may have the same risk factors as patients with stroke, but so far this connection has not been determined. In the New York Stroke Data Bank, certain factors seemed to correlate in those with both stroke and dementia: specific kinds of large-artery atherosclerosis, advanced age (seventy years or more), and the presence of more than one stroke. Obviously, further investigations will be critical if we are to determine the risk, the risk factors, and the causes of dementia in patients with stroke.

Conclusions

Because people in our society are living longer, physicians, particularly neurologists, will be seeing a larger number of patients with dementia. This trend will certainly continue in the immediate future. Dementias resulting from disorders of the aging brain are expected to increase through the remainder of this decade and probably the next one. Epidemiology plays a crucial role in determining diagnostic standards, disease characteristics (natural history, distribution and frequency measures, and predictor models), risk factors, and outcome measures and is the basis for evaluating treatment.

The health service needs of the elderly will increase, but the exact nature and scope of expansion are unclear. Uncertainty about financing health care and programs for the elderly has limited how physicians can plan for this "neurological burden." Changes will be required at all levels in the health care system, from basic medical education to the delivery of services.

The federal response to this pending crisis has been adequate, and we as clinicians must keep that momentum going. Geriatric training centers, grants for research on Alzheimer's disease and related disorders, and the establishment of Alzheimer's disease research centers and centers for the investigation of psychopathology, or psychological and behavioral dysfunction, in the elderly have greatly focused investigators. However, day-to-day problems, such as financing extended care in hospitals and nursing homes, have limited the amount of enthusiasm we have about the federal support of these programs. Faced with the possibility of an aging population, many of whom may be part of an epidemic of astounding proportions, our efforts must continue at full pace. We may have to extend Lewis Thomas's designation of Alzheimer's disease as the "disease of the twentieth century" into the next hundred years, unless the twenty-first century brings about advances in the treatment and an understanding of the causes of disabling neurological diseases of the elderly.

Suggested Reading

Robert N. Butler, "The Life Review: An Interpretation of Reminiscence in the Aged," *Psychiatry* 26 (1963), pp. 65–75.

Robert N. Butler and Myrna I. Lewis, *Aging and Mental Health* (3rd ed.). Columbus, OH: Merrill, 1986.

Robert A. Nemiroff and Calvin A. Colarusso (eds.), *New Dimensions in Adult Development*. New York: Basic Books, 1990.

Joel Sadavoy and Molyn Leszcz (eds.), *Treating the Elderly with Psychotherapy: The Scope for Change in Later Life*. CT: International Universities Press, 1988.

III

WHEN SPECIAL HELP IS NEEDED

15

Health Care of the Elderly

A Nurse's Perspective

THELMA J. WELLS, R.N., PH.D., F.A.A.N., F.R.C.N.

Introduction

"The unique function of the nurse," writes a distinguished nursing leader, "is to assist the individual, sick or well, in the performance of those activities contributing to health or its recovery (or to a peaceful death) that he would perform unaided if he had the necessary strength, will or knowledge. And to do this in such a way as to help him gain independence as rapidly as possible."[1]

This core definition of nursing supports the specialty of gerontological nursing, which is characterized by dynamic, pragmatic actions aimed at helping the older person achieve and maintain the level of physical and social functioning appropriate to his or her individual lifestyle and environmental needs.

Some years ago, I challenged that

> the nurse in gerontology must demonstrate excellence in nursing care, communicate knowledge and methods to help other nurses achieve such excellence, become a change agent in the health care system for the improvement of services to the elderly, and become an active partic-

> ipant in scientific inquiry, interdisciplinary professional care teams, and community affairs related to the needs of elderly people.[2]

Since, then, significant advances have been made in the nursing care of the old.

In this chapter I briefly review nursing as a field and gerontological nursing as a specialty. I then focus on specific practice areas: acute care, nursing homes, home care, and mental-health–psychiatric illness. Across these practice areas, I have identified common areas of grave concern: education, reimbursement, ethics, morale, and leadership.

The perspective is from current nursing practice in the care of the elderly. The direction is toward collaborative interdisciplinary exchange, the unique feature of the National Academies of Practice. The goal is the development of an action agenda for the academies.

Nursing

Nursing as a professional field has continued to evolve from its recent birth in the nineteenth century. Currently, there are three quite different educational paths, all leading to the registered-nurse licensing examination. The oldest of these programs is commonly called the *diploma*. Based in hospital nursing-education departments, diploma schools constitute 14 percent of the current basic nursing programs. The newest education offering is the associate degree, based in community colleges and constituting 53 percent of the available programs. Baccalaureate nursing education in colleges and universities has been available since 1909 and makes up 32 percent of programs.

The goal of nursing leadership across more than six decades is to move nursing preparatory education to only two entry levels: the professional, prepared at the baccalaureate level, and the technician or assistant, prepared at the associate degree level. Specialization in nursing occurs at the master's degree level; continued expansion is evidenced by a 15 percent increase in such graduates between 1986 and 1987. Overall, about 6 percent of employed registered nurses (RNs) have a master's degree. There are currently forty-five doctoral programs in nursing with a consistent increase in enrollments and graduates. About .3 percent of employed RNs have a doctorate.

Slowly but surely, a transition is taking place in nursing education, but as in any transition, confusion may result. This is especially compounded in nursing by the unfortunate use of the term *nursing* in a generic sense, as in *nursing home.* It is interesting that other professions have been able to avoid generic terminology. In the health care field, there is no analogous confusion with doctoring and social working, for example. However, the central point is that the term *nurse* needs to be clarified in any discussion. For a start, is the reference to a registered nurse or another level of worker? And if to a registered nurse, what educational background is consistent with the role requirements?

Recently, a crisis in nursing has been affecting health care. "The reported shortage of RN's is real, widespread, and of significant magnitude," writes the Secretary's Commission on Nursing.[3] Hospitals, which employ two-thirds of RNs, reported a doubling of RN vacancy rates between 1983 and 1987; 76 percent of hospitals reported RN shortages, 19 percent considering this shortage severe. Thirty-four percent of nursing homes report a severe RN shortage. The RN shortage seems to arise primarily from a greater demand for increased technical, complex, and cost-effective patient care. Of great impact on the shortage is a continued decline in combined enrollment figures for preparatory nursing programs, with a fall of 13 percent between 1983 and 1985.

Gerontological Nursing

This background about nursing education in transition and critical shortage in the field sets the context for a discussion of nursing care for the elderly. In 1966, the American Nurses' Association established a Division of Geriatric Nursing, later renamed Gerontological Nursing. Growth in the specialty over the last three decades has been rapid and significant. Over four thousand nurses have been certified in gerontological nursing by the American Nurses' Association. Given the 1.5 million RNs employed, this seems like a very small group, but certification is still a new and evolving process in nursing. Key points to note are that gerontological nursing is a recognized specialty with an educational base, certification processes, and a beginning political voice.

To give a picture of the health care of the elderly from a nursing perspective, a process combining a literature review, field interviews, and personal experience was followed.

Acute Care

The acute-care hospital has always been characterized by a fast tempo, but the effort to limit rising health costs through the implementation of diagnosis-related groups (DRGs) has increased the tempo. In a short view of acute care, DRGs have been successful. The average length of stay in nonfederal short-stay hospitals for those sixty-five and over declined by a full day between 1983 and 1985. The central obsession of hospitals has become survival in the health care industry. This obsession is not always consistent with safe care, ethical care, or quality care—goals that are seldom spoken of these days.

My local newspaper reported the need for one thousand nursing-home beds in our region by 1993; they were needed to alleviate "bed backup" in local acute-care hospitals. "Bed backup" is caused by "geriatric and certainly chronically ill patients, many of whom don't need acute hospital care."[4] Such patients are labeled as needing an alternate level of care (ALC). The September 1989 figures for my county listed 467 such patients, averaging 131.6 hospital days; about 25 percent of these patients held beds in emergency rooms.

Hospitals have become high-tech centers where the elderly are supposed to be whisked in and out. What do you think the care atmosphere is like for someone classified as not belonging, keeping a bed from those who really need it? As high-tech, fast-paced settings, acute-care hospitals find it increasingly difficult to meet the time requirements of rehabilitation, or even standard care, for older people. Consider the pace and needs in light of a critical nursing shortage. I seriously wonder if the term *care* fits what happens to elderly people in acute-"care" settings.

A clinical nurse specialist in acute care remarked that she thought the major issue in her hospital was education. Noting that care of the elderly was not a standard requirement in nursing education, she reflected that in-service education programs had been significantly curtailed by the work load; there was no time for staff nurses to attend programs. A major focus of her job was a project to reduce patients' length of stay. The project was fraught with poor measurement, questionable assumptions, and naive design, but it showed length of stay decreasing for the elderly, so it was continued as part of the hospital's data bank. One wonders if the time spent gathering the questionable, if not meaningless, data might have been better spent.

Regulations within this hospital itself seemed to curtail certain types of care for old people. For example, the criteria for admission to the rehabilitation unit, in effect, rejected the majority of old people in the hospital. Discharge planning, a hospital priority for old people, was beset by internal communication issues as well as external restraints. For example, maintenance physical therapy at home was not covered by Medicare. Help with instrumental activities of daily living, such as shopping and laundry, was also seen as essential.

"Everything is short-term," the clinical nurse specialist said about health insurance. "There is no coverage for chronic needs, and most elderly with some financial resources are afraid to spend these for fear that, if in the future they need a nursing home, they won't have adequate sums to get one of their choice."

Nursing Homes

Nursing homes. These days that is where the elderly go to reduce the length of their acute hospital stays. One DRG study in Indianapolis showed that, although the average hospital stay had decreased from 16.6 to 10.3 days, discharge to nursing homes had increased from 21 percent to 48 percent, and even six months after discharge the proportion of patients still in nursing homes had increased from 13 percent to 39 percent.

The problems in nursing homes used to be gigantic; they are now colossal. As a nursing director told me, "Bureaucratic regulation is now more pervasive, less reasonable, less logical, and more costly." As an example, she presented some of her experience with the Omnibus Budget Reconciliation Act (OBRA) of 1987. One requirement of the act is for a national data base.

The federal model was a six-page tool. New York State is now piloting a twenty-six-page tool with eight to nine pages to be completed by physicians ("Who do you think will end up gathering those data?" the nursing director asked, implying that similar data requests of the past had been, in fact, fulfilled by nurses); three to four pages to be completed by social workers; and the rest, about twelve pages, to be completed by the nurse. This tool is to be completed for all admissions—quarterly—and when a patient's condition has changed (a state currently undefined). This substantive data base, added to the already substantive documentation required, would appear to effectively bury nursing-home nurses under paperwork.

The director cited yet another good idea gone bureaucratic from the OBRA 1987 requirements: All nurse aides in long-term care must be registered. This mandate came with no guidelines and a rapid implementation date. Directives addressing aide registration seem to arrive weekly with requests, changes, or revisions as everyone struggles with this mammoth task. She calculates that, in her large facility, 1.2 full-time RNs have been used on this requirement so far. Such time was not budgeted for and thus takes away from other planned nursing functions.

It is essential in discussing nursing homes to consider how much professional nursing is available in them, especially when such nursing is increasingly directed toward documentation, as in the examples noted. Overall, only about 7 percent of registered nurses are employed in nursing homes, but how many, if any, are in a facility varies considerably. Less than 6 percent of nursing homes are required to have an RN on all shifts. Just over half the nursing homes in the country (51 percent) have no state minimum full-time RN requirement. In addition, the nursing-home RN spends less time per patient per day, as compared to an RN in a hospital. Given the limited number of RNs in nursing homes, it is not surprising that less than 10 percent of their time is spent in direct-care activities. In fact, the two most common activities of nursing-home RNs are assigning and supervising staff and observing and charting patients, the latter also called *documentation*.

Yet, the basic-care and rehabilitative needs of patients in nursing homes are staggering. A third need help eating; almost half have a problem with bowel or bladder control; a third are chair-bound; almost a third need assistance with walking; and 69 percent need help dressing. The goal of nursing-home care has got to be more than minimal custodial service. With DRG imperatives pushing patients into nursing homes, these settings must become sophisticated and expert rehabilitation facilities.

Home Care

"It is no secret to any nurse in community health care that the DRG system has caused major shifts in the nature of the patient load, types of patients served, and level of care technology required," writes a research team studying the home care issue.[5] Nurses in home care now have larger patient loads, with more patients who are acutely ill and in need of complex care services.

Declaring home care in a state of crisis, the director of the New York Visiting Nurse Service (VNS) writes, "The rules governing reimbursement of services grow more complex and their application more unpredictable."[6] She chronicles the interaction of federal, state, and city home-care rules and regulations as they affect her agency. One gets the sense that everything is in flux all the time, that there is no dialogue between the different regulating agencies, and that there is no piloting, planning, or even reasoned discussion between the regulating agencies and the service providers.

Among health professionals in this field, I hear and see morale at a new low. Conscientious people are leaving, and the recruitment of professionals into the care of old people seems more of a problem than ever. The NAP should be a catalyst to revive the spirit of professionals who care for old people. Through the recognition of quality service, as in awards and the promotion of positive programs through media exposure, the special advantage of the NAP's reach across the professions can be highlighted. The focus on mutual support rather than territorial conflict can strengthen the resolve to continue to work toward quality health care for old people.

Leadership. We seem to be in an era when it is not popular. Whether the leadership deterrent is fear of litigation, of loss of votes, or of threats to physical survival, the outcome is a dismal morass in the status of the health care of old people. The future does not gleam bright.

Yet, almost because quality health care is so obviously struggling and perhaps going down for the count, the time is excellent for a new kind of leadership. The National Academies of Practice should move into the breach and provide united, coordinated action plans to address the health care crisis. The dream of the NAP holds great promise: to step beyond the confines of all disciplines and link with other colleagues as, together, we provide the direction for quality, ethical, and cost-effective care.

Notes

1. V. Henderson, *The Nature of Nursing*. New York: Macmillan, 1966, p. 15.
2. T. J. Wells, "Nursing Committed to the Elderly," *Current Practice in Gerontological Nursing*, ed. A. Reinhardt and M. Quinn. St. Louis: C. V. Mosby, 1979, p. 190.
3. Secretary's Commission on Nursing, *Final Report*, U.S. Department of Health and Human Services (July 1988), Washington, DC, p. 2.
4. M. E. Arch, "'1,000 Nursing Home Beds Needed by '93,' Report Says," *Times Union*, January 4, 1990.

5. E. K. Phillips, M. E. Fisher, D. MacMillen-Scattergood, and A. J. Baglioni, "DRG Ripple and the Shifting Burden of Care to Home Health," *Nursing and Health Care*, 10:6 (1989), pp. 325–327.
6. E. I. Griffith, "Home Care in Crisis: Turning It Around," *NO*, 36:6 (1988), pp. 272–274.

Suggested Reading

American Nurses' Association, *Facts about Nursing*. Kansas City, MO: The Company, 1987.

Division of Nursing, *The Nursing Shortage: Facts, Figures, and Feelings*. Chicago: American Hospital Association, 1987.

Division of Research, *National Data Review*, National League for Nursing, New York, 1989.

16

Geriatrics

Recommended Approaches to Averting a Crisis in Care

SANDRA MACKAY, R.N., PH.D.

Introduction

Because of the unprecedented changes that are taking place in the age structure of American society, profound changes will need to occur in many of the health and social systems that have a direct impact on the elderly. In this chapter, I briefly review some of these trends and make recommendations about how nursing can help to avert a crisis in long-term care of the elderly in the coming decades. As we have begun to realize, this goal will mean shifting from hospital-oriented care to community- and home-based care and placing greater emphasis on promoting a high quality of life rather than merely extending life.

Making More Selective Use of Hospitals

Although hospitals are only one facet of the health care system, since World War II such acute-care facilities have dominated the health care scene—and often the landscape around them as well. Many hospitals, particularly teaching hospitals, have prided themselves on having the most advanced forms of medical technology that can be found anywhere in the world and have adjusted rewards and prestige accordingly. This attitude has not only fostered competition between hospitals but promoted deep division within them. Essentially, the medical system has become one in which the "in" group gets most of the resources and works with inpatients, while those who are "out" work with outpatients.

Although this pattern is gradually changing, many physicians and nurses who were trained before the 1980s still have difficulty shifting gears from acute illness and episodic care and tend to overlook the preventive and rehabilitative aspects of patient care. There is also an overreliance on inpatient treatment and a tendency to use such settings for terminal patient care, when other options might be more appropriate.

Part of the answer to reducing the escalating costs of health care in the United States will be to make much more selective use of hospital services in the 1990s. Currently, a bed in an American hospital costs anywhere from several hundred dollars a day for one on a general medical-surgical floor, to well over $2,500 a day for a bed in the intensive-care unit of a major city hospital.

An equally important reason for making a more selective use of hospitals is that the ideology in these settings makes it very difficult for physicians and nurses to stop treatment and allow a patient to die. When disease is still seen as a battle to be won, the death of a patient is often equated with defeat. This stance may produce "heroic efforts" to keep patients alive at all costs. Although such efforts are needed to reverse acute, life-threatening conditions, they merely prolong the dying process for those whose diseases have progressed so far that they are irreversible.

The inevitable questions that arise when many of these efforts seem fruitless or increase a patient's suffering usually include: Why couldn't he have been allowed to die in peace instead of putting him through all that? When should treatment have been withdrawn? And why wasn't there a "no-code order" (a "do-not-resuscitate" order signed by the patient's physician) in the patient's chart?

This growing concern among health care providers about what can be done to prevent elderly patients from having to endure what are often traumatic and undignified ways of dying provides nursing with a wonderful opportunity to begin working with other professions to develop more caring alternatives that will be acceptable to both patients and providers. Through such existing structures as ethics committees, discharge planning conferences, and quality assurance programs, it may be possible to improve the terminal care of seriously ill patients and to create a wider range of community care options for the elderly in the future.

Reducing the Disproportionate Use of Health Care Resources

Such collaboration is urgently needed so that older people will not continue to consume such a disproportionate amount of the nation's health resources. In the mid-1980s, Americans over the age of sixty-five constituted only 11 percent of the population but purchased 25 percent of all prescription drugs, were admitted to 40 percent of all acute-care hospital beds, received over 50 percent of the $80 billion allocated to health in the federal budget, and accounted for roughly 33 percent of the total $287 billion that was spent on health in the United States. Moreover, $25 billion (28 percent) of the entire Medicare budget was spent on terminally ill patients during their last year of life.

The Nurse's Role in Reducing Health Care Costs

For nursing to meet its responsibilities in containing costs, we need to free our thinking and begin exercising a leadership role in developing policies that will transform how health care is delivered. Let us consider, for example, one of the ways in which hospital nurses can improve the care of terminally ill patients without additional funds. Currently, it is up to the physician to inform a patient about a terminal illness as well as any options that are available for palliative treatment. Very often, the nurses who are taking care of the patient are not told what the physician has said to the patient, and nothing about this discussion is recorded on the chart. This lack of information makes it very difficult for nurses to provide the supportive care that the patient needs and to deal as effectively as they would like with the psychological distress of family members.

Because nurses are the ones who are with patients most of the time in the hospital, it is important for such professional issues to be discussed more openly so that physicians and nurses can begin working toward joint practice policies that will improve patient care. Then, instead of having to be evasive when patients question nurses about their illness, the nurses will be able to respond to the patients' and family members' concerns.

Policies should also be changed so that a nurse caring for someone who is terminally ill can discuss the options for care that are available at home through various community nursing services. For instance, hospice home-health programs assist families in caring for dying patients, and visiting-nurse agencies often provide twenty-four-hour services for a wide range of seriously ill patients, including those who can be relieved of severe pain through surgically implanted pumps that dispense morphine or who are on parenteral therapy (prolonged intravenous therapy for nutritional support through venous access devices) because their nutritional reserves are severely compromised.

Hospital nurses should also be able to inform terminally ill patients and their families of the possibility of withholding or withdrawing life-sustaining measures in a hospital or nursing home. Many elderly patients would be greatly relieved to know how they can be cared for without being hooked up to machines. Unfortunately, in our present youth-oriented culture, physicians are still apt to downplay the true nature of a bad prognosis. Patients are often not told that they are terminally ill until they are too sick or incapacitated to fully participate in the decisions that are made about their treatment. Thus, the life-sustaining care being given the ten thousand patients currently being maintained in what is considered a "persistent vegetative state" may not be in accord with their previously stated wishes.

Wider Use of a Durable Power of Attorney for Health Care

A much better way for many Americans to begin dealing with these issues would be for nurses to take a leadership role in providing them with information about a "durable power of attorney for health care" before they become too sick or mentally incapacitated to understand such an option. Statutes have been enacted in all of the states to enable a durable power of attorney to become effective and remain effective whenever the person who initiates it becomes incompetent and another person is needed to manage his or her property. Fourteen states also allow separate durable powers of attorney for health care. Nurses could introduce similar health legislation in the remaining states and educate the public about the advantages of a durable power of attorney for health care, which is more comprehensive than a "living will" or a "directive to physicians." This legislation would enable people to learn more about artificially prolonging life when there is no hope of recovery from an accident, a chronic condition such as an irreversible coma, or an end-stage disease. They would also learn why they may want a document that becomes effective as soon as it is needed, rather than only when death is imminent and they have been diagnosed as terminally ill. A durable power would also enable patients to select the person they would like to make health care decisions for them if they become unable to do so for themselves, to give that person access to their medical records, and to specify the kinds of medical interventions that they want and do not want. Because a durable power also continues in effect after a person's death, timely decisions about such things as donating organs can also be made, in accordance with the patient's wishes.

Such actions by nurses would be in keeping with the Patient Self-Determination Act that went into effect on December 1,

1991. Under this law, nursing homes, hospitals, home health agencies, hospices, and prepaid programs such as health maintenance organizations are required to provide information and education about such advance directives to patients, staff, and community members in order to continue receiving Medicare reimbursement.

As such legally binding documents become more widely used by the elderly, health care providers will have clearer guidelines when patients become incapable of making health care decisions for themselves. These documents also make it possible for an older person's loved ones to know how much intervention the patient really wants if there is no reasonable likelihood of his or her recovery. This knowledge will prevent many of the conflicts that occur between family members when they are faced with such critical decisions during highly stressful times.

Practicing within the Upper Limits of Training

Nursing services are vital in meeting the health care needs of older Americans. But if the most effective use is to be made of this health care resource, it is essential for nurses to function at the upper limits of their training more of the time. Nurses are being taught in school to perform physician examinations on their patients, yet they are not being encouraged to use these skills if they work as staff nurses in the very hospitals and clinics where they have been trained. Nor are they likely to be reimbursed for these skills in many nursing homes and community health settings. Even nurse practitioners and nurse clinicians, who have received additional medical preparation, often find that many of their skills are ignored or downplayed by the organizations in which they work and that advanced clinical roles have not been integrated into the daily work of their units and departments. Frequently, head nurses and administrators are as reluctant as physicians to acknowledge the clinical expertise of nurses, and the nursing notes may be so physically separated from the rest of the patient's record that they are not noticed by other professional groups, whose own clinical findings have been better integrated into the record.

To maximize the nursing resources that are already available in many hospitals will require not only organizational support from the top down but support from other departments as well, if nurses are to discontinue performing such nonnursing tasks as delivering trays, obtaining medication from the pharmacy during nights and weekends, transporting patients, and carrying out various secretarial tasks.

The prospect of having enough money to pay for the health care of older Americans would be much better if some basic reforms were made in other support services as well. For example, the medical record system in many teaching hospitals frequently operates in such a way that patients must be seen by providers who do not have ready access to the patients' records. These records are available on inpatient units, but not in the outpatient department. Thus, nurses in each clinic begin to develop their own systems of recording and storing their records. Although information flows vertically to the central medical-record room, it does not flow horizontally to nurses in the other clinics where the patient is seen. Thus, it is almost impossible to coordinate care, and services may be duplicated.

Increasing the Levels and Sophistication of Nursing Care

Methods of reimbursement for patient care will also need to be modified in the future to reflect the increasing levels and sophistication of nursing services that are needed by the elderly in order to ensure them continuing access to high-quality care. Although the idea for diagnosis-related groups (DRGs) originated with a nurse, it was originally intended to classify medical and surgical conditions for epidemiological research, not to classify the patient in general. Nevertheless, DRGs have become the major system for classifying medical and surgical conditions for reimbursement purposes, even though they do not provide an accurate indicator of the level of nursing care that patients require.

Often, elderly patients are admitted to a hospital because of the amount and type of nursing care that they require. As soon as the acuteness of their illness decreases, patients who required beds in an intensive-care unit can be transferred to another hospital setting where there are fewer nurses for each patient and less sophisticated technology. The level of nursing care is also a crucial factor in ambulatory care. By 1996, it will be possible to do more than 60 percent of all surgical procedures in an ambulatory setting. Which operations are performed in outpatient settings will largely depend on the amount of postoperative nursing care required. It is essential, then, that whatever reimbursement systems are used in the 1990s be indexed to the intensity of nursing care required and that patients be treated in the settings that are most appropriate for their needs.

Patients who are hospitalized in the future will be seriously ill and will require the most technically sophisticated nursing services that can be provided. Those who are discharged to their homes may well need even more follow-up nursing services than they do at present. Unfortunately, there is a shortage of nurses and decline in those enrolling in nursing programs, in contrast to the excess of physicians and built-in incentives for increasing the number of procedurally oriented subspecialists (e.g., cardiologists, gastroenterologists, radiologists, cardiovascular surgeons, and orthopedic surgeons).

Given the high costs of educating nurses and the number of years involved, an increase in nursing personnel might be achieved more readily if we had scholarship or financial aid programs in our universities that would lend nursing students money for their education and living expenses. In return, the recipients could pay back loans with a small, tax-deductible percentage of their salaries during the years that they practice their profession. This plan would enable more men and women to go into nursing and would reduce the need for so many nursing students to complete their education on a part-time basis while supporting themselves with jobs in other fields.

Enough funds would be available to staff night, evening, and day shifts more adequately if less money were paid for simple medical procedures and some of the routine operations that are performed. The continuing practice of overpaying for services that do not require much intellectual effort or a high level of manual skill and underpaying for services that require a great deal of both obviously enters into decisions that students make in choosing professional fields, and it may be partly responsible for the increasing popularity of foreign medical schools and the decreasing number of applicants to collegiate nursing programs. Once one can practice a surgical specialty, it is relatively easy to increase the number of surgical procedures that are performed in the community where one lives. Indeed, the rates of relatively simple surgical procedures, such as hysterectomies and tonsillectomies, depend more on the practice patterns of the local physicians than on any characteristics of the patient population. Therefore, it is time for more rational decisions to be made about how many surgeons the nation should produce over the next few decades and what other kinds of health workers can do to prevent a crisis in health care for the elderly.

Taking a More Proactive Stand to Improve Health Care

At present, we devote most of our effort and health care dollar to reacting to diseases that already exist, when what is needed for the future is a system that is much better at preventing disease and disability, or at least delaying it, and that is far more proactive in nature. For example, one of the most poorly funded areas of health care is the public health system. Yet, improvements in sanitation were largely responsible for many of the improvements in the health of Americans earlier in this century. Public health nursing has also distinguished itself by the successes it has had in teaching people how to adopt more healthy lifestyles and can point to many achievements in this area, particularly in regard to the early recognition and control of tuberculosis, diabetes, glaucoma, hypertension, polio, and many sexually transmitted diseases, including human immunodeficiency virus (HIV). But they cannot continue some of these efforts in the 1990s, much less expand them, without substantial increases in funding for public health programs.

If our health insurance systems rewarded a more proactive approach by nurses, we could reach out to many more groups in the population and prevent much of the disability that plagues people throughout their lives. For example, health screening by nurses in schools and public health agencies could ensure that orthopedic problems, visual defects, hearing loss, and speaking problems in children would be picked up early and corrected in their earliest stages. Health teaching of older children and adolescents by nurses would also decrease the number of teens who get pregnant, would reduce the spread of sexually transmitted diseases, and would help to ensure early prenatal care for teens, who are among those most likely to deliver low-birth-weight infants with their associated medical problems. If nurses used their physical-assessment skills to screen older patients for the retinal changes associated with diabetes, these changes could also be picked up much earlier, and patients could be referred to an ophthalmologist for treatment that would delay or prevent blindness. This service would obviously help to promote more independent living for older people, as they would be able to continue activities that would be difficult, or even impossible, with further impairment of their sight.

If younger adults were reached earlier through periodic screening examinations before they became ill, we might be able to reduce much of the disease that is now associated with aging, such as heart disease, cancer, and stroke, and to achieve significant cost savings over time. Theoretically, further reductions in morbidity and mortality could be brought about by providing more financial incentives (e.g., significantly reduced insurance premiums) for those people who changed their habits and adopted more healthy lifestyles, such as stopping smoking, exercising more regularly, eating healthier, more low-fat and high-fiber diets, and continuing those practices that have been shown to be beneficial, like avoiding the use of drugs and wearing seatbelts. In 1979, the U.S. Surgeon General reported that more than half of all the deaths that occurred in the United States could be traced to inappropriate behaviors or unhealthy lifestyles.

Although we are just beginning to see the outlines of the health care system that will become possible in the information age, it is clear that advances in technology can make health services more convenient for patients. As an example, cardiac changes lend themselves particularly well to being monitored over long distances. This approach is already being used by nurses to check pacemakers that have been implanted in older people. Similarly, pregnant women who are in danger of going into premature labor can be monitored over long distances by specially trained obstetrical nurses who have expertise in fetal monitoring. This use of new technology saves money because patients can be cared for at home rather than in a hospital, and it enables the treatment of many more patients at a time. In the case of fetal monitoring, it can also prevent many of the lifelong disabilities associated with prematurity. An expanded use of new types of technology may enable many other types of patients to be treated at home in the future.

Efforts to keep people well should also include a wider use of prospective payment systems by large corporations and an increased use of nurse practitioners. Prepaid health-insurance systems have a tremendous advantage, as medical expenditures can be budgeted for well in advance, and the total costs of these services can be fixed while the contracts are in effect. However, these health services not only must be managed so that they are cost-effective but must be structured so that professionals can provide care in a way that is acceptable to patients.

The largest health maintenance organization (HMO) in this country, and one of the most sensitive to the needs of its patients, is the Kaiser-Permanente Medical Care Program, which served 3.9 million people in the late 1980s. Physicians at Kaiser saw a need to provide more affordable care to large numbers of people, who often had to wait a long time for their clinic appointments, so the program added nurse practitioners to the staff because there was a shortage of physicians. Although there is now an oversupply of physicians, Kaiser has continued using nurse practitioners because they save a lot of money, improve access to care, have fewer malpractice suits, maintain excellent relationships with patients, and save about 70 percent of a physician's clinic time. Studies of nurses who practice in these settings indicate that they achieve excellent patient care outcomes with fewer tests than physicians tend to use. They also put more emphasis on teaching patients what they need to know to manage their diseases effectively at home.

Reducing the Need for Nursing Homes

In keeping with a more proactive stand, nurses need to question the wisdom of adding a lot more beds to nursing homes when these homes are often no more than warehouses for the elderly. Many senior citizens prefer services that will allow them to live in their own homes. Often, nursing homes charge well over $100 a day for what amounts to just room and board. There are additional charges for medications, medical equipment, and personal services, such as laundry, as well. Because many are private facilities, run with the intention of making as much money as possible, the ratio of registered nurses to patients tends to be very low, and most of the care that the residents receive comes from practical nurses and attendants. Physical therapy, speech therapy, and other therapies are seldom provided to more than a very small proportion of the patients.

Research has shown that the likelihood of being admitted to a nursing home is more closely related to the availability of a spouse, or someone else at home, than to the physical condition of the patient. This fact is important because, even though the media perpetuate an image of older couples living out their golden years together, in reality only about 3 percent of those who marry when they are young are still together for their fiftieth wedding anniversary. Some spouses die, of course, but an increasing number of older men and women are also choosing to divorce. Since the early 1970s, the divorce rate among older men and women has risen three times faster than the rate of growth in this population. Remarriages do occur even late in life; however, the likelihood of having a spouse in old age is much greater for men than for women. According to the 1986 U.S. Census figures, 70 percent of the men who are seventy-five and older were married, in contrast to only about 24 percent of the women of this age. Because women live longer than men, once they are admitted to a nursing home they may live there for a long time. After a few years in such an institution, virtually no one is discharged back into the community.

The risk of institutionalization is particularly great for those who are alone, so nurses need to be aware that 8.3 million people in the age bracket of sixty-five and older lived alone in 1988; 25 percent of them had no living siblings, and 8 percent had no siblings or children who were alive. Data from four years earlier indicate that older people with at least two living children were less likely to be living alone than those with only one child alive. What is clearly needed to prevent more people from being admitted to nursing homes in the years ahead is a wider range of nursing and related services that will make up for the care that families are unable to provide.

Vastly expanded home health and social services—help with grocery shopping, housekeeping, and transportation; more outreach vans for preventive services; elder day care to help younger family members who work; and numerous other services—could be rapidly expanded through the efforts of nursing organizations, business groups, and churches. Excellent models for meeting the health needs of particular subgroups within the population are available in some of our cities. For instance, On Loc meets a wide variety of nursing and housing needs for elderly men and women who live in San Francisco's Chinatown. In the Japanese-American community, Kimochi, Inc., has organized health and nutrition programs for seniors so that they include the youth and promote strong intergenerational ties within the San Francisco Japanese-American population. Similarly, work by the San Francisco AIDS Foundation, public health nurses, and a myriad of community agencies has enabled a large number of terminally ill patients to be cared for at home. Earlier, it would have been considered impossible to create such a vast network of services in a community in such a short time.

Care-giving responsibilities for a patient who wants to be allowed to die at home require more than managing the disease process. The work that the nurse does can extend beyond the patient's life to being the one to pronounce the patient dead, helping the spouse or partner make funeral arrangements, and then providing follow-up visits for bereavement counseling.

Centers for Extended Nursing Care

Long-term facilities will always be needed for patients who cannot be safely managed at home, or who require monitoring and care around the clock. But we need to be sure that any patients "with chronic illnesses who are unable to carry out their usual activities, or who are at risk of suffering serious complications but who have the potential to return to independent living"[1] do not end up in these beds. One of the best hospital-based extended-care programs has been the Loeb Center at Montefiore Hospital and Medical Center in New York City. This program is administered, directed, and conducted by professional nurses, with physician consultation from the medical center, and is both patient- and family-oriented.

Since the late 1960s, the Loeb Center has consistently demonstrated its efficacy in reducing hospital readmissions, and in reducing the related costs for the elderly while improving their functional abilities. This program allows nurses to use the full range of their knowledge and skills, and the result is high job satisfaction among the nurses who work there.

Long-term nursing centers that deliver high-quality services to groups of severely incapacitated geriatric patients could be set up along the same lines as the Loeb Center and could be designed and equipped specifically for this level of nursing care. Few existing nursing homes have the equipment required for complete nursing care. The design of some actually increases the work load of the staff. For instance, if a neurologically impaired patient could be weighed or moved into a chair by one nurse with the assistance of a lifting device, but three or four staff members have to do the job because there is no way that this piece of equipment will fit next to the patient's bed, then the room is poorly designed for such patient care.

Model centers for long-term nursing care, such as I am proposing, could be developed in conjunction with the Veterans

Administration (VA) as a means of improving care for the elderly in a relatively short period of time. The VA already runs the largest health-care system in the country and, for a number of years, has had hospital-based programs that are administered by nurses. It also supervises the care of many elderly patients in community board-and-care home, has a geriatric research capability, and provides care to a geriatric population that is already experiencing many of the changes that the rest of the society will face two decades from now. Moreover, the VA predicts that men and women over seventy-five years old will need four times more nursing-home beds than patients who are ten years younger, unless the present health-care-delivery system is changed.

Fortunately, the VA is in an excellent position to modify the traditional ways of delivering care because it is already affiliated with medical and nursing schools throughout the country and serves as a clinical education site for several other professional groups. With some changes in its accounting practices and an influx of talent from major business schools, the VA could also be used to develop techniques for accurately predicting the costs of the services required by the most dependent segment of the elderly population. This prediction would provide realistic guidelines for reimbursing the private sector for comparable services in the future.

Although such competition with the private sector may be resisted, it would be feasible in view of legislation that already exists. In 1970, Public Law 91-50 expanded the eligibility for health care benefits to all U.S. veterans over the age of sixty-five, regardless of their ability to pay. Although many men and women who are eligible for VA services still use the private sector for their health care, more will be turning to the VA in the future as out-of-pocket costs begin to outstrip their ability to pay for care they need.

If the VA were charged with developing model centers for long-term nursing care and were given enough targeted funding to do the job right, it might be able to concentrate more of its research, teaching, and practice in this area and achieve outstanding results within a decade or so. This progress would enable the VA to meet many of its own goals as well as those of the larger society. However, time is running out, and we need a lot of work in this area to develop the programs that are needed to meet society's responsibilities to its oldest citizens.

Ensuring High Quality of Health Care for the Elderly

The Teaching Nursing Home Program, co-sponsored by the Robert Wood Johnson Foundation and the American Academy of Nursing, has already demonstrated the feasibility of changing patterns of practice in nursing homes through collaboration with professional schools. However, to upgrade care in the future, it will also be necessary to pay more realistic salaries to nurses who work in this health field and to implement staff-to-patient ratios that promote a quality of care that the staff can be proud of. Nurses and others who have chosen to work in nursing homes are often dedicated to caring for older patients and want to do a good job. Although there are some bad apples in this field, just as there are some bad attorneys and bad physicians, people are more likely to treat those who are dependent on them well when they are being treated well themselves.

Cost containment in health care is certainly possible, as I have indicated, but if it is to be very effective and is not to lead to even greater turmoil in the years ahead, we must understand how the current system functions. We have already seen what happened when the back wards of our mental institutions were closed without our having an effective network of community-based mental-health services in place or enough low-cost housing for the chronically mentally ill. Such older men and women can hardly be considered better off sleeping in public parks, eating in soup kitchens, or foraging for food and clothing in garbage cans, regardless of how much money was saved by the closing of these institutions. If we do not want to repeat such experiences in the future, we must redesign our health and social systems so that we have the programs we need to care for much larger groups of elderly patients in the years ahead.

In the next section of this chapter, I describe some of the trends that may occur in the lifestyles of older men and women. In doing so, I also point out why I believe that, in order to be successful, health care policies will have to be planned in collaboration with the elderly.

Developing Policies That Promote the Welfare of the Elderly

An area that is often overlooked in the education of nurses is how the political system works in relation to special-interest groups, such as older Americans. Although these men and women seldom vote as a bloc, they have the potential to do so when the issues are of as direct concern to them as those in health care, and they also use their voting rights much more frequently than young people. Older citizens tend to vote in higher percentages than those who are younger. It is anticipated that the issues that the country will face in the twenty-first century will draw even more older voters into the political process.

The idea that politicians of either party know what is best for the elderly was challenged several years ago when catastrophic-health-insurance legislation was introduced in Congress. Although there was input and support from the largest group representing the elderly, the American Association for Retired People (AARP), there were no large-scale surveys by the professions to find out how particular subgroups of the elderly felt about this legislation or thought it should be financed. When the legislation was passed, the resulting uproar among senior citizens at the grass-roots level caught both health workers and politicians by surprise and resulted in some fast backpedaling on the part of Congress. Not only did older Americans question the need for catastrophic coverage, when many wanted better chronic-disease and home-health coverage, but they also resented the Medicare program's reaching into their pockets without their consent. The legislation was repealed.

Older Americans Are a Diverse Group

It is often assumed that older Americans constitute a rather homogeneous group. The reality is that there is as much diversity in ethnic composition, political orientation, religious affiliation, and various other characteristics as in any other subgroup. There are also remarkable variations in the way people age and when this aging seems to take place. Some artists have been highly creative very late in life and have produced outstanding work well into their eighties. Other octogenarians can perform physically strenuous activities, such as the Triathlon, acrobatics, or chopping wood. Academic achievement is also possible for some very old people, as demonstrated by a woman who completed her associate-in-arts degree at the age of 104.[2] Now that so many older Americans are alive in the eighth and ninth decades of life and may even live much longer in the next century, it is important for nurses to expand their knowledge about how healthy aging takes place.

Managing Transitions Well

By studying the lives of elderly people who manage various transitions well, who are healthy in old age, or who excel in particular areas, nurses will learn what may be possible for many more people in the twenty-first century and will be in a better position to develop methods of practice that promote physical and mental well-being throughout the life span. A number of excellent techniques for encouraging patients to present their life stories as they see them, embedded in the rich context of their own cultural and ethnic traditions, already exist in the social sciences and could be readily adapted for use by nurses to learn more about the way patients face challenges late in life.

Such stories are needed if we are to begin to see older men and women as they really are instead of as our TV shows would have us see them. For example, significant transitions such as having one's children leave home or retiring from a job may be looked forward to with great pleasure by some couples and with considerable dread by others. Both the empty nest and retirement may put intense pressure on relationships, and couples who are facing such transitions may need counseling from nurses to make these changes successfully. This is not very surprising, as all societies recognize that there are certain transitional periods in the life cycle in which old roles are given up and new ones are taken on. The resulting changes in status are difficult for most people unless society provides some mechanisms for helping them get through these passages.

Support Systems

If we study the support groups that have sprung up to help people cope with the death of a loved one, the isolation of caring for a spouse with Alzheimer's disease, or the changes in roles that take place after a stroke or some other disabling condition, it is possible to learn a great deal about the capacity of humans to adapt to change late in life. Telephone support systems for elderly people may also yield valuable information about the strategies used by people who live alone.

Many live on small pensions in single rooms in hotels that are in the seediest parts of town and must go elsewhere for all their meals. Outreach work by public health nurses is needed to reach homeless elderly men and women, often former residents of mental institutions, who move from shelter to shelter and may have to sleep in a doorway or walk all night to avoid the dangers of the streets. We know very little about this population, including what preventive health services they need and how to provide these services in a way they will accept.

Living Benefits

Insurance benefits can also be redesigned to promote the welfare of the elderly. For example, the Prudential Insurance Company of America announced a new life insurance policy that would permit certain policyholders to qualify for what are called "living benefits" or accelerated death benefits if they are terminally ill. This policy enables patients to collect the benefits that would have accrued after death—minus some interest on this money—during their last six months of life if they are living in a nursing home for six months with no prospect of leaving, or if they live elsewhere but have a doctor's certificate stating that they are not expected to live longer than six months. Other plans penalize policyholders for withdrawing their money early by charging them stiff penalties.

At this writing ten states have approved this plan. New York's insurance laws prohibit accelerated death benefits; Connecticut allows them only for long-term care in a nursing home; and many other states prohibit them on the assumption that it would be too confusing for consumers if life insurance benefits were not kept clearly separated from health insurance benefits. Not only is this attitude patronizing, but it is also unwise to limit accelerated death benefits to those in nursing homes. Only about 5 percent of the men and women who are sixty-five and older live in nursing homes; most live in communities. Thus, such laws may actually promote more costly forms of care in the future. Although Prudential's life insurance policy gets around this problem by allowing payments to those in non-nursing-home settings, it does require a physician to certify that the patient has not more than six months to live. This requirement seems unnecessarily restrictive, as there is no sure way for physicians to predict who will live for six months and who will live somewhat longer.

Reverse Mortgages

Encouraging banks to offer their clients reverse mortgages is another creative way for nurses to assist elderly clients who want to remain in their own homes but have very little money. Through this practice, older persons do not have to sell their homes to meet their living expenses. Instead, the bank agrees to buy the house back, and the person receives the money from the reverse mortgage in regular monthly payments for as many years as it takes for the bank to purchase the property. This plan is very acceptable to many families who would otherwise have to sell the house and move. However, studies have shown that if legislation were passed to accommodate more reverse mortgages, and if the general public learned more about the benefits of this idea, as many as one-fifth of the nation's elderly poor could move above the poverty line and remain in their own homes.

Retirement Communities

For those older men and women who can afford it, there is a great variety of retirement communities to choose from. Some do not allow children as residents; others are multigenerational. There are also life care communities that provide a wide range of nursing services, including nursing-home care, as well as various types of residential complexes that provide no health programs at all. For the 30 percent of the elderly who live alone, a retirement community may be particularly attractive because it provides numerous opportunities to make new friends, many recreational facilities, and safe living quarters. Some require that older people purchase their living units, with the stipulation that after they die their units will revert back to the retirement community. Others allow the sale of residential units that people no longer want.

Matching Roommates and Shared Housing

Retirement communities are not for everyone. Matching roommates and sharing houses or apartments is another option for nurses to suggest to older people who do not want to live alone. Boston's Shared Living Project, started by the Gray Panthers and several churches in a remodeled mansion, provides a home for both young and very old adults. This type of living arrangement has been so well received that there are now hundreds of similar programs around the country that are sponsored by churches and other community groups. With nursing's support, this number could grow much higher in all areas of the country.

Influencing the development of health and social policies is an important part of being a professional. It requires an understanding of the problems that are likely to be faced within the foreseeable future and a willingness to grapple with tough issues, on which it is unlikely that reasonable people will always agree. To keep pace with the enormous changes that are taking place in American society, nurses will need to be able to draw on knowledge from a wide range of disciplines. Joint master's and doctoral degrees may become more common in the decades ahead, and nursing facilities may have to share personnel to get the expertise they need for their programs. Eventually, there may be so much overlap between nursing and other fields that new disciplines will have to be established and/or some of the weaker fields absorbed by the stronger ones.

There are very few guideposts for health workers to follow in educating their young, as no one has ever lived in a society where so many men and women live as long as they do now. But we can learn more about the services that each of our professions can offer society in meeting its responsibilities to its oldest citizens, and we can set some reasonable goals that we can work together to achieve.

For older patients to get the nursing services that they will need in the years ahead, nurses must work with other professional groups to establish the patient-to-staff ratios in hospitals, nursing homes, and home health agencies that are essential for adequate patient care and specific enough to be incorporated into national accreditation procedures. Thus, nurses will have to give up tasks that should be done by others, and to take steps to make sure that the unique services that professional nurses provide are visible to others.

Paying for Nursing Care in the Future

To achieve many of the goals I have outlined, nursing should work with physicians and other professional groups to limit the amount of money that can be collected in malpractice suits. As we all know, high settlements seldom improve care for other patients and only drive up the price of health care for everyone by promoting "defensive medicine" on the part of physicians.

We will also need to work together to ensure adequate national funding for health care in the future. We should consider the possibility of having a basic national-health program for pregnant women, infants, and young children. The value of early prenatal care has been well established as a low-cost method of reducing the number of low-birth-weight infants who are born in a community. Such infants are at much greater risk of dying during their first year of life, and if they live, they may have health problems that will significantly impair them for the rest of their lives. Providing health care to infants and young children also makes sense when one recognizes that a person who benefits from good health care in infancy and early childhood may be able to live another seventy-five years as a productive citizen. Such a basic insurance plan could be more like a Chevrolet than a Cadillac, so we could phase in other groups within the population as these children grow up, if that seemed feasible.

By keeping more people healthy and treating diseases much earlier, we can avoid many of the long term costs associated with a large elderly population. In the year 2040, there will be eighty-seven million Americans over 65, and by 2080, around five million people will be over the age of 100. As our population grays, there will be fewer young people in the work force to support each person who retires and draws a Social Security check than there are at present. In 1935, over 40 workers contributed to the pension of each person who received a Social Security check; in 1990, there were only 3.4. By the year 2020, the support ratio is expected to drop to 1.78 workers for each retiree.

The prediction of such a sharp decline in the tax revenue base leads many to question the future solvency of these trust funds and the strength of the medical safety net for the most vulnerable members of our society. Congress amended the Social Security Act in 1965 to include hospital treatment and home care services for the elderly (Medicare), and to assist the states in expanding health services for the indigent (Medicaid). The funds for Medicare programs are derived from three sources: Social Security payroll taxes, general federal revenues, and direct charges to enrollees through premiums and policyholders' copayments. Part A of Medicare is particularly important to nursing because it covers hospital costs, some skilled nursing, and limited home-health services. Thus, the future viability of many nursing programs that provide direct patient care may be in jeopardy if there are fewer funds to pay for these services in the future.

Part B of Medicare is a voluntary, supplemental medical insurance program that pays for physician services, outpatient care, some medical equipment, and certain home-care services. There would also be an impact on future nursing programs if its revenues decreased, particularly because all Medicare programs provide health insurance coverage for anyone who is eligible for Social Security without regard to income. This group includes young disabled people who meet the criteria for eligibility as well as most older people in the United States. The future solvency of Medicaid funding is also crucial to nursing. This program enables individuals who are so poor that they have to be on welfare to receive care in hospitals, from home health agencies, and in long-term-care facilities.

Even though neither Medicare nor Medicaid reimburses nurses or other providers for services at their full rates, federal expenditures for these two programs have soared in recent years, and expenditures for Medicare are expected to increase each year. The costs of Part A of Medicare will begin to exceed its revenues from payroll taxes and these funds may be totally depleted by 2002; hence a key source of revenue for many nursing programs will not be available. Part B of Medicare will be less of a drain on the Social Security system because it receives 75 percent of its funding from general tax revenues and 25 percent from premiums paid by enrollees.

The Medicare and Medicaid budgets could be strengthened by a combination of strategies that would decrease costs and increase revenues. Nursing would play a pivotal role in this process, as I have indicated, because it can help to decrease the costs of caring for the elderly both now and in the future. This kind of decrease would be more feasible than trying to increase revenues through taxation, as there is a limit on how high taxes can be raised, and trying to raise the age at which Social Security benefits will be paid may be difficult.

Reductions in Medicare and Medicaid coverage would also hurt millions of people who have benefited from one or more governmental programs. Social Security and Medicare are presently the two most heavily used programs. If health insurance benefits in these programs are cut, there is little likelihood that many elderly people could pay for nursing care themselves.

The financial circumstances of middle-class people would change drastically if they became seriously ill or required long-term care for a chronic condition and had less insurance coverage. Even though the elderly tend to have more discretionary income than those who are younger, this would not begin to cover the costs of caring for anyone with a heart attack or cancer.

Summary and Recommendations

Perhaps the greatest challenge for nursing in the 1990s is to change the mission of the health care system from reacting to disease that already exists to the more proactive stand of preventing disease and disability and teaching people how to adopt healthier lifestyles. This approach has long been advocated by the nursing profession, but it is particularly important now because it would reduce some of the diseases that are common in the elderly.

Several recommendations for achieving this goal include expanding public-health-nursing programs to include more preventive services for groups of elderly people, including those at risk of being admitted to nursing homes; expanding supportive services for older people who need some assistance with grocery shopping, transportation, and housekeeping in order to continue living in the community; and using nursing and other services to rehabilitate patients rather than warehousing them in nursing homes.

To enable more people to live at home, we should also promote the wider use of reverse mortgages and should work with older men and women to develop new living arrangements, such as shared housing and matched roommates for those who do not like living alone.

Other supportive services that are needed to help elderly people who want to continue living in the community, but who have various kinds of limitations in their functional abilities, include day treatment centers, as well as numerous health and social services that are provided through visiting-nurse and home-health agencies.

In urging the nursing profession to work with other professions to establish standards that can be tied to national accreditation procedures for staff-to-patient ratios in hospitals, nursing homes, and some health agencies, I hope to establish goals for improving patient care that we can work toward together. Nurses can play a pivotal role in reducing health care costs if they are permitted to practice at the upper limit of their training more of the time, that is, if they give up nonnursing tasks and make full use of their professional resources.

To rapidly improve the long-term care of the elderly and to teach health workers how to deliver health care services in new ways, we need to establish a substantial number of centers for long-term nursing care around the country. To accelerate the process, it is suggested that the Veterans Administration be given the major responsibility and the financial resources to develop model programs that will demonstrate how high-quality nursing care can be provided cost-effectively to large numbers of elderly men and women. Such model programs not only should serve as clinical-training and research sites for teams of health workers who need to learn new ways of delivering care to the elderly but should also be used to furnish the kind of data that will be needed in the future to guide federal reimbursement practices for comparable services.

To provide the range of nursing services that will be needed by the elderly in the decades ahead, it will be vital to restructure payments so that routine medical procedures and operations are reimbursed at lower rates. This reduction would help to ensure that we will not continue to produce more procedure-oriented specialists than the nation needs. To reduce the duplication of tests and services will require support services that function in ways that enable nurses to coordinate care no matter where the patient is seen. It is also suggested that nurses work with other professionals to limit the amount of money that can be collected in malpractice suits, as large settlements seldom improve care for other patients and drive up the costs of health care for everyone.

To decrease the costs of terminal care, nurses need to promote policies that expand the use of durable power of attorney for health and to create additional options for using life insurance benefits before death. We also need to expand hospice programs, along with other alternatives for care at home, and to discuss options, such as the withdrawal or withholding of life-sustaining measures, before patients are too sick to participate in decisions about their own care. The ability to discuss these options will require joint practice agreements with physicians and policies that ensure that nurses will have the information that they need to work more effectively with terminally ill patients and their families.

The provision of nursing services for large numbers of older Americans will require substantial improvements in how health insurance is paid for in the years ahead. With the predicted shortfalls in Medicare funding, the gains that many senior citizens have made in health care in recent decades could be virtually eliminated.

To strengthen the medical safety net for all of us as we age, strenuous efforts are needed to increase revenues and to decrease the costs of health care services. Some of the solutions may be special taxes on cigarettes and alcoholic beverages that are specifically targeted for Medicare programs; a much more selective use of hospitals and nursing homes; an increased use of nurse practitioners; and phasing in a basic national-health-insurance program starting with pregnant women, infants, and children that would ensure a healthy start for the next generation and prevent many of the neurological deficits that have disabled others throughout their lives.

By setting our sights on where we want to go as a profession in meeting our responsibilities to the elderly, we may be able to avert a crisis in long-term care in the twenty-first century.

Notes

1. G. Alfano, "Hospital-Based Extended Care Nursing: Case Study of the Loeb Center," *Nursing in the 1980s* (1982), p. 211.
2. H. Mather, "An Overview of the Veterans Administration and Its Services for Older Veterans," *Older Veterans* (1984), p. 34.

17

Social Work Services for Older People in Acute or Long-Term Care

BARBARA BERKMAN, D.S.W. AND
ROSALIE A. KANE, D.S.W.

Introduction

The elderly, those sixty-five and older, represent approximately one-tenth of the U.S. population. If current trends continue, this percentage will grow to 21.2 percent by the year 2030; the proportion of the "older-old" (seventy-five and older) is expected to rise most dramatically.

Older people, especially those over seventy-five, are generally at risk of suffering limitations in their ability to perform activities of daily living (ADLs), such as dressing, bathing, using the toilet, transferring in and out of bed, and feeding themselves. Many experience urinary incontinence as well, which has severe implications for daily functioning. They are also more likely to be limited in the instrumental activities of daily living (IADLs) associated with independence, such as cooking, cleaning, laundry, communication by telephone, driving or other transporting of themselves, shopping, and the management of money. Services that compensate for such ADL and IADL impairments tend to be labor-intensive and expensive. Receiving such services demands many social and psychological adjustments for older people and their families.

Often, decreasing function is associated with severe and chronic illness, which frequently increases with age and places the elderly at greater risk of dependency than younger populations. There may be a decrease in resources and the availability of family assistance which, in conjunction with more illness and dependency, causes increases in the admissions of the elderly to hospitals and nursing homes.

Although only 5 percent of persons over sixty-five reside in nursing homes at any given time, the chance that people who survive to age sixty-five will enter a nursing home before their death is better than one in four. In part, the high use of nursing homes is attributable to the limited availability of affordable or publicly subsidized home care. For every nursing-home resident, two equally impaired people are living in the community. Most of these manage with family help and minimally paid or free home care.

Both medically oriented and socially oriented services for functionally impaired older people in their own homes have expanded since the early 1980s. The older person's need and ability to be maintained at home requires careful assessment in light of his or her family and social situation. Social workers, sometimes bearing the title of *case manager,* have been called on to conduct comprehensive assessments of the older person's physical, psychological, cognitive, and social functioning; to allocate home care according to a care plan that is acceptable to the older person and the family; and to carefully weigh the risks and benefits of home care in their recommendations.

Currently, 30 percent of hospitalizations are now devoted to care for the elderly, who are frequently admitted for longer stays and are generally in need of treatment for multiple conditions. In addition, elderly frail patients are at high risk for recurrent admissions to the hospital because of the severity of their illnesses, their age, and the impact of psychological and social stressors on the disease course and recovery. Almost one-fourth of Medicare inpatient expenditures are for readmissions that occur within sixty days of discharge. It has been estimated that readmissions account for almost half of all hospital admissions and 60 percent of hospital charges. Readmission costs range from 24 to 55 percent higher than first admissions.

Admission to the hospital not only is costly economically but also takes its toll physiologically and psychologically on the elderly and their families. Older persons are acutely aware of their body's increased vulnerability due to chronic functional disability, which frequently leads to major life changes. Elders who experience the disruption of a hospitalization may also have heightened fears of loss of physical health and increased dependency on family members. It is understandable that they may react to being hospitalized with anxiety and fear, which cause additional stress on their physiological system.

These stressors increase the risk of the patient's becoming confused and disoriented and therefore less able to the manage postdischarge care necessitated by the disease. When the patient's capacity to comply with medical recommendations is compromised, the likelihood of a repeat hospitalization increases. These patients are considered "high-risk" individuals who need extra services from social workers in making the transition from the hospital to posthospital care, whether in their own homes or in other facilities. Moreover, with ever shorter hospital stays and the tendency to discharge older people for brief recuperative stays in nursing homes, short-term nursing-home residents need extra services from nursing-home or other community social workers.

In recent years, the interaction between psychosocial processes and recovery from medical illness has been a topic of professional research as well as of popular discussion. The severity of the illness and the common risk factors alone (e.g., hypertension, exercise, smoking, weight, and alcohol consumption) have failed to predict the general disability of many elderly patients. Several studies have looked toward a broad range of psychosocial and demographic variables to account for the differences found in recovery outcomes. The growing body of literature supports the contention that the existence and interrelationships of multiple psychological and social factors interact with functional capacity to affect the occurrence and severity of many illnesses, general disability, and recovery from the illnesses. In other words, the course and outcome of severe illness may well be affected by psychological and social as well as physiological variables. The disease, the individual's ability to cope and adapt, family involvement, and social networks all interact and affect the illness.

In this chapter, we explore those variables, or combinations of variables, that, when interactive with physiological factors, significantly relate to recovery, risk of death, and other outcomes, such as entering a nursing home. We often focus here on cardiac patients, one major group that has been helped by social workers and on which considerable amounts of data are available. By doing so, we hope to illuminate the factors that should be considered by social workers in their interventions with elderly patients.

The research base for understanding the effect of psychological and social variables on outcomes for elderly persons has been developed largely in hospitals. Our review touches on other sources of data when possible, but there are few longitudinal studies that track older persons who have used mixtures of acute-care and long-term-care services over time.

Psychological Factors

Numerous studies have focused on psychological factors as they relate to recovery outcomes. The available reported research on causative psychological factors is not definitive because research in this area is very complex. However, there is beginning evidence relating psychological variables and recovery, and the importance of psychological stress factors in recovery after heart attack has been well established. Often correlating with each other, these factors may influence the recovery process and prognosis. Further, a marked increase in the emotional stress of myocardial infarct patients has been reported after discharge from the hospital. Although normal, these reactions may have a negative impact on prognosis.

It is not unusual to react with depression, anxiety, and denial when experiencing a major life event. These three psychological factors have been identified as relating to problems in the recovery of elderly patients and to their subsequent readmission to the hospital. Depression and anxiety have also been identified among older persons needing long-term care. Typically, older people have deep-seated fears of entering a nursing home and also dread the loss of control involved in accepting services in their own homes.

With long-term care, the focus of concern also embraces relevant family members, many of whom are over age sixty-five. Husbands and wives, adult children (often themselves retired), and siblings may experience depression, anxiety, and anger because of the burden involved in giving care at home. Sometimes, too, the older person needing care may have priorities and preferences that differ from those of family members. Some data suggest that older people fail to discuss these preferences with their responsible family members and that they often make no plans for declining health and functional status.

Depression

The depression that many cardiac patients experience is well documented in the literature. It has been suggested that almost three-quarters of patients are significantly depressed for one year following the onset of a heart attack. Some feelings of depression are universal, appearing most often around the third or fourth day after the acute crisis has passed.

The presence of depression has been identified as a negative factor in recovery. For example, depression following myocardial infarction (MI) is a major barrier to rehabilitation, inhibiting the patient's ability to follow medical regimens. Stress of a relatively mild nature has been reported to be capable of causing problems in physiological recovery among cardiac patients, and emotional upset immediately following an MI has been correlated with delays in the resumption of full activity.

Studies show that depression is more predictive of negative recovery outcome and readmission than is the severity of the infarct. Patients depressed at their first posthospital visit have been found to be at risk of a negative outcome, and those who do not survive have shown a high rate of prolonged depression.

Anxiety

The hazards of extremes of anxiety in recovery have also been studied. Several studies have found that anxiety was positively correlated with depression, and that depressed patients, especially women, had more readmissions and higher six-month mortality rates than those who were not depressed. Female MI patients are more likely to display anxiety than men and are more often readmitted to the hospital. Emotional distress also results in a less satisfactory recovery in terms of personal adjustment and returning to work.

Studies that have examined the effect of psychological reactions to MI have found a significant reduction in the mortality rate of those patients who received help in dealing with their anxiety and depression. Those patients treated for psychological reactions had shorter hospitalizations and tended to develop fewer complications.

Denial

Several studies have explored the impact of denial on recovery. Denial has been defined as a repudiation of part or all of the total meaning of an event in order to minimize or reduce anxiety. Whether denial is protective or maladaptive appears to depend on when it occurs. Denial is present at three stages in the course of a disease: during the prehospital onset of symptoms, during coronary-care-unit (CCU) treatment, and during short- and long-term recovery.

Denial during the onset of symptoms may be maladaptive if it delays medical care. It has been found that 12 to 20 percent of patients repudiate the illness or the need for treatment. During CCU care, denial can lower anxiety and increase rates of survival; 20 to 80 percent of patients repudiate feelings of fear, anxiety, or apprehension during their hospital stay. Denial here may be a positive force, as it has been found to be related to reduced in-hospital mortality and faster recovery. The continuation of denial during recovery is maladaptive if it interferes with compliance with smoking cessation, rest, diet, and reductions in work schedules. On the other hand, it has been reported that deniers return to work earlier, remain employed at one year after MI, resume sex with less difficulty, and report fewer physiological and psychological symptoms.

Thus, denial is a factor that may have both negative and positive implications for the patient. When it defends the patient against anxiety, it may be positive therapeutically, allowing the patient to participate better in treatment. It may also give elderly cardiac patients a feeling of predictability and control over their lives that is related to positive outcomes during recovery. Increasing the parent's behavioral as well as mental control may lead to a decrease in the harmful side effects of stress as well as of other feelings of distress.

On the other hand, denial may be maladaptive if it results in a delay in the recognition and treatment of cardiac symptoms or in noncompliance with medical advance or in expectations that are too high or too low for a person's capabilities.

Social Support Factors

Another dimension that is significantly correlated with morbidity and mortality, independent of physical health status, is social support: family, friends, and community resources. Social support "encompasses the emotional support, advice, guidance and appraisal, as well as the material aid and services that people obtain from their social relationships."[1]

A number of writers have studied the patient in relation to his or her social context. Social support has been found to maximize adaptation and coping and also enhances self-esteem and self-control. When social support acts as a buffer against stressful life events by reducing physical and psychological breakdown, it is a significant predictor of recovery from MI. Maintaining social networks has been found to be related to lower rates of hospital admission and readmission and to be beneficial to recovery. Thus, social support has a direct effect on health status. Positive social support, in particular, is salutary for both health and well-being.

Lack of social support and feelings of loneliness have been correlated with illness, disability, and higher mortality rates. Social isolation and high stress, independent of physical risk factors, are significantly associated with greater risk of cardiac death. Many authors suggest that the family members' knowledge about the elderly patient's illness and treatment during the recovery period and their ability to cope with the stress of post-hospital care influence the recovery outcome of the patient. If elderly cardiac patients, once discharged, are isolated from any kind of social support (e.g., the workplace, friends, professional health-care workers, and neighbors) or family (e.g., spouses, children, and extended family), or if they encounter negative family reaction to their health state, their emotional response may lead to an early readmission.

The ability of patients to resume productive work lives has been found to be a significant measure of recovery outcome. Failure to resume work is associated with increased levels of emotional distress. If one is able to work after a myocardial infarction, he or she appears to recover and do much better, regardless of the severity of the infarct, than those patients who, because of age, gender, occupation, socioeconomic status, or job dissatisfaction, are unable to return to work.

Marital status as a specific dimension of social support has been studied in relation to survival after an acute myocardial infarction. It has been found to have a positive influence on in-hospital and long-term survival rates in a number of studies. Among elderly cancer patients, those who were severely ill and living with their spouses were less likely to be at risk for long-term institutionalization; however, they were more likely to be rehospitalized. These authors speculated that rehospitalization may be used as a form of respite care for family members.

However, not all social support has positive effects. Excessive family attention may lead to greater disability and failure to return to work, either by family members' doing too much for the cardiac patient or by their verbally discouraging activity.

Also, conflicts among family members during cardiac recovery are not infrequent.

One study found that long-term care of a chronically ill family member results in too many expectations placed on the caregivers. As the situation grows less tolerable, the caregivers may protect themselves by using distancing behavior. Thus, though few impaired elderly are abandoned by their families, strain increases with the chronicity of the illness. The elderly experience a drop in morale and an increase in feelings of loneliness as the quality and quantity of caregiving become more perfunctory.

Research is beginning to explore the link between social networks, events in the social environment, and the development of chronic heart disease. However, one should be cautious about drawing conclusions concerning the absolute relationships of social networks and disease causation. To guide research, the concept of social support needs to be more precisely defined and measured within a theoretical structure or model.

Sense of Control as a Factor in Recovery

Closely related to social support is the patient's sense of control. Researchers have found that a sense of control influenced the outcomes of MI patients more than illness severity, prognosis, preillness stressful life events, and social support measures. Although it is unclear whether a sense of control leads to better outcomes or whether medical improvement leads to an increased sense of control, the significance of this factor should not be ignored. It would seem that a person's sense of her or his capacity to effectively respond to problems depends on the nature of her or his social supports. That is, family members who engage their elderly cardiac relative in decision-making processes, as well as societies, communities, and households that are supportive of and conducive to independent functioning (provide, e.g., old-age income, grocery delivery services, and downstairs bathrooms), enhance the perceived sense of control. Those that do not significantly impede it.

For the elderly patient, who is often asked to follow special diets, take medication and adhere to an exercise program, a sense of control may also be associated with the ability to comply with the recommended regimens. In order to facilitate compliance, it is useful to quantify such instructions as "Don't over exert." Greater compliance often occurs when instructions are written down for patients. It is suggested that these measures prove successful, in part, because they enhance the cardiac patient's capacity for control.

The phenomenon of learned helplessness, first described in animal models, has been observed particularly among older long-term-care users, particularly nursing-home residents. It is characterized by dwindling efforts to influence the environment, depression, and an eventual failure to perceive when one has had an effect on the environment. Learned helplessness has been associated with increased morbidity and mortality among nursing-home residents and among persons on waiting lists for nursing homes. Experiments conducted to increase perceptions of control have had positive outcomes.

The literature on relocation is more ambiguous because of the difficulty in controlling for health status. Evidence indicates that, when older persons perceive that they have not chosen to move to a new living setting, such as a nursing home, and when the life in the new location cannot be predicted to be similar to their previous patterns, psychological and physical regression may occur.

Functional Risks

Impaired capacity in basic activities of daily living (i.e., ambulation, eating, personal hygiene, and control of bowel and bladder) are functional problems that imply that the individual will have a more difficult time adapting to illness and will have a higher need of home assistance or long-term institutional care. Self-perceived functional disability is also associated with higher rates of morbidity and mortality in cardiac patients.

Many elders suffer functional problems that interfere with

recovery from illness and that may require special adjustments and services. Sensory deficits such as blindness or partial blindness contribute further to functional impairments and difficulties in performing the activities of daily living. Other sensory impairments, such as hearing deficits, which are extremely common among the elderly, may exacerbate any cognitive difficulties present. Cognitive problems, with accompanying memory loss, also affect recovery.

Many of the conditions affecting older people bring functional impairment in their wake. Stroke, arthritis, hip fracture, congestive heart failure, and chronic pulmonary disease, such as emphysema, are associated with mobility problems, generalized weaknesses, and an inability to perform both basic and instrumental activities of daily living. Dementing illnesses, such as Alzheimer's disease, and their associated cognitive loss also lead to functional disability. Because functional disability may be the result of interacting physical problems, iatrogenic effects of treatment, cognitive problems, and/or emotional problems, the clinical challenge is to adequately disentangle the causes of the functional impairment, to correct the correctable, and to eliminate any "excess disability," that is, any disability beyond that warranted by the condition.

As this older population continues to increase, more patients will be at high risk for posthospitalization complications in recovery and will suffer early recurrent admission. We can expect, then, more need for home social-health-care services. Estimates vary between 9 and 50 percent that readmissions can be prevented by improved medical care and follow-up, better monitoring of medication for adverse reactions, better patient compliance with treatment, and better home supports.

Social Work in Hospitals

The health-care social worker generally sees older hospitalized patients at a point of crisis. These patients are out of their normal settings, temporarily sick, and wishing to return home. They may have limited physical and intellectual powers and are likely to be experiencing depression and feelings of helplessness, and to feel resentful and frightened.

The current illness may be only the latest expression of many physical problems, inasmuch as illnesses tend to be more frequent and longer lasting in the elderly than in younger persons. The patient is also dealing with many life changes that may engender loneliness, boredom, and the fear of growing old. Contributing to these changes are the aging of the older person's peers and the death and infirmity of family and friends.

Although most older people have at least one child who lives within a very short distance, geographic mobility may mean that some children and many friends have moved elsewhere. At the time of hospitalization for a serious illness, out-of-town children often converge and attempt to make plans in an atmosphere of crisis and haste, sometimes with tensions arising between the out-of-towners and the local relatives. Social workers can be helpful in defusing the sense of crisis, assisting family members in planning, and ensuring that the elderly patient will not be left out of the decision making.

Discharge Planning

Discharge planning is one of the tasks that social workers are frequently called on to perform. More clinical skill is required than is often recognized. In the health care system, the social worker works with the inpatients and their families during periods of stress usually associated with an illness, the development of a disabling condition, or the exacerbation of a physical handicap. The intervention provided is an outgrowth of the worker's assessment of the client's difficulty and need. There are five states in the discharge-planning process: assessment, diagnosis, prescription, implementation, and evaluation. A major role of the social worker is to explain and manage the psychosocial elements of patient care as they pertain to discharge planning.

Approximately 50 percent of social work clients in hospitals are elderly patients. With a frail elderly population, an important part of effective social work in health care practice involves planning for social, psychological, and environmental supports. Patients, and the family members involved with them, need support to find ways of adapting both to the specific illness and to the long-term implications of increased disability. The first few weeks at home following an initial hospitalization are of critical importance.

Early identification of those patients most likely to be negatively affected during posthospital recovery by psychological, social, and functional stressors is essential so that professionals have the time, while the patient is still in the hospital, to arrange for the necessary posthospital social and health services. These services, in turn, should minimize the chances of early recurrent admissions, which may result from breakdowns in the patient's support system.

Social workers are looking for valid ways to identify early those patients in need of posthospital care. The ability to target posthospital services for those high-risk individuals may have a strong impact on improving social health-care delivery and reducing premature rehospitalization. The identification and refinement of high-risk factors is a necessary first step toward the development of a screening mechanism that will identify such high-risk patients.

Another important component of discharge planning is assisting patients to plan for their future needs at a time of stress and crisis. Many do not plan for crisis and therefore are unprepared for the posthospitalization period. Other factors that interfere with successful posthospital-care planning have been identified as a lack of adequate posthospital resources such as extended-care beds, the limited cooperation of medical staff in the necessary paperwork, and the changing medical condition of the patient.

Social workers traditionally work directly with patients and develop and advocate for programs that ensure access to continuous quality care. An emerging role for social workers is assisting patients to exercise the amount of control they desire over the discharge plan. A recent study revealed variations in the amount of control patients desired. Patients with an internal locus of control and thus a desire to make decisions experienced high levels of stress when they perceived they had no control over the discharge plan. For many elderly patients, participating in the discharge-planning process may have a positive impact on posthospital recovery.

Medical Decision Making

As medical technology makes it increasingly possible to prolong the life of very ill patients, difficult decisions arise daily in hospitals regarding whether life-prolonging procedures such as cardiopulmonary resuscitation and the use of ventilators should be started or stopped for a particular patient. Some states allow living wills and durable powers of attorney for health, and some older people give advance directives permitting the withholding of treatments or empowering an agent to make decisions in their behalf.

Research is gradually beginning to explore the extent to which family proxies and older people would agree on decisions in hypothetical cases. In practice, however, even with advance directives, end-of-life decision making is rarely clear-cut, and the process is extraordinarily stressful. Social workers will be increasingly called on to assist older people and their family members in clarifying the alternatives and achieving comfort with their decisions.

Social Work in Nursing Homes

The nursing home is an arena where social workers can play pivotal roles in helping the resident to live as meaningfully as possible. They can develop programs and routines in the nursing home that are compatible with autonomy and dignity for the residents. The importance of the latter has been documented in studies that show that cognitively intact nursing-home residents deplore their lack of control and choice over their everyday life. For those residents who are about to leave the nursing home, social workers can help bridge the gap between the nursing home and the community by making well-thought-out discharge plans.

Although models exist for skilled social work in nursing homes, until recently the presence of social workers in nursing homes has been minimal. With new requirements enacted in 1987, a full-time social worker is required in all nursing homes that exceed 120 beds. As a result, social workers have the opportunity and challenge to fully develop practice in the nursing home, and to help ensure that a good quality of life will be maintained and that residents' rights will be observed.

Social Work in Community Long-Term Care

Many community-based long-term care programs are funded by federal and/or state programs. Social workers are increasingly involved in the allocation of the services offered by these programs, including home care, chore services, adult day care, home-delivered meals, and transportation. Often, the social worker is considered a case manager, whose job includes identifying the patients in need of help; making a comprehensive, multidimensional assessment; planning care; arranging services; monitoring the cases and reassessing the case. Case managers are challenged to be advocates for the particular client while also distributing resources fairly and effectively.

The research focusing on case management is now at a descriptive stage only. For example, it is known that many older persons would rather refuse home care or accept lower levels than they need for their safety than enter a nursing home. Case managers must recognize that older persons range in their risk levels. They need to determine how to weigh the wishes of an older person and at the same time take into account the protection of their safety and community safety. In the next decade, the social work practice of case management will, we hope, become refined on the basis of data about the outcomes experienced by patients receiving long-term care at home.

Future Trends

The health care industry now faces tighter fiscal controls at the federal, state, and local levels as well as increasing scrutiny by the private insurance sector. Alternatives to inpatient hospital care are being sought, and new, expanding ambulatory-care services are becoming the norm.

For social workers to remain a vital part of the emerging health-care programs, they must be innovative in their approaches to patient care. Efficiently developing and executing discharge plans for patients will continue to be the most significant role of hospital social workers. Social workers in community long-term care, such as home care services, must be innovative in their approaches and may be increasingly involved in case management. Social workers working in long-term institutional care must help residents to live as meaningfully as possible by developing programs that support their autonomy and dignity.

Note

1. K. Ell, "Social Networks, Social Support, and Health Status: A Review," *Social Service Review* (March 1984), pp. 133–149.

Suggested Reading

Barbara Berkman, "Social Work in Health Care: A Review of the Literature," American Hospital Association Catalogue #187902. Chicago: American Hospital Association, 1988.

R. A. Kane and R. L. Kane, *Long Term Care: Principles, Programs, and Policies*. New York: Springer, 1987.

18

Practitioners as Consumers of Services for the Aged

FLORENCE LIEBERMAN, D.S.W.

The National Academies of Practice, the sponsor of this symposium, requires that an individual who is designated as a Distinguished Practitioner have fifteen or more years of practice which must include outstanding contributions to practice excellence. As a result, the members of the National Academies of Practice tend to be on the older side of the age spectrum and are either personal consumers of services for the aged or have family members—a spouse or an elderly parent—who needs various health services. Therefore, this summary focuses on two facets of health care and health needs: the feelings and needs of the consumer and the concerns of and directions for the health professionals who provide these services.

Aging in Good Health

Though being older does not mean that one is ill or disabled, as people are living longer than ever before changes in abilities are inevitable sooner or later. For example, one Distinguished Practitioner has two parents about eight-five years old who, until recently, maintained their old family home. Because of professional demands, their children had moved to other parts of the country. The parents began to accept limitations in their ability to care for the large house, which they no longer needed, and driving at night was becoming more difficult, curtailing their attendance at the concerts and plays that they enjoyed. Additionally, they were feeling the loss of most of their contemporaries and were in need of social contact with others for talking, bridge, and golf. In consultation with their children, they sold their home and entered a retirement community. Here, there were people, some with major disabilities, who were all a potential source of interaction. In addition, transportation was available when needed. For their children, there was the security of knowing that, if illness occurred, care was readily available.

Recreational programs in senior centers, Y's, churches, schools, colleges, and other community groups provide opportunities for socialization, education, and trips, as well as, frequently, nourishing and inexpensive meals. Some of these centers also provide some medical checkups. A growing number of housing developments that have been established for the older family are organized to provide similar opportunities; some retirement communities enable their residents to live in individual apartments and at the same time oversee some of their needs, which may include meals and emergency and medical care. All of these enhance the quality of life of the elderly and assist in maintaining a sense of integrity and purpose.

Aging and Illness

The major source of stress for older people and their families is physical illness, particularly when it is accompanied by any disability that entails dependency on others. However, many problems of the older years can be prevented by early detection and prompt remediation, which require regular examinations and regular care. For example, periodic eye examinations can detect changing vision needs or the early emergence of other problems. One hundred percent of the elderly require some form of vision care, which is provided by optometry or ophthalmology. For many, optometry is the primary entry point into the health care system. Though there is an optometrist in over 90 percent of the counties in the nation, vision care is the second largest unmet national health-care need of the elderly.

Regular podiatric visits can prevent foot ailments that curtail physical activities and frequently target the beginning symptoms of diabetes. Prevention of immobility is possible through devices and treatments that are less costly than the consequences of neglect. Yet the reimbursement policies that determine how the elderly receive care encourage the development of problems that could be prevented in the long run and contribute to the rise in the health care costs of the nation.

Regular dental checkups help maintain healthy gums and prevent the loss of teeth; however, only 35 percent of the elderly seek dental services. In addition, regular and complete physical examinations will detect the beginning of problems that can be prevented or at least alleviated. None of these is reimbursed by Medicare. As a consequence, too many elderly people do not use health services before an acute need arises.

In addition, some elderly individuals who are still in good health and vigorous may feel that regular examinations are not necessary, particularly if the habit of regular checkups has not been a part of their lifestyle. For others, cultural conflicts, illiteracy, or the inability to speak English may interfere with an understanding of the essential value of preventive care.

In any case, the amount of paperwork that has to be completed and the difficulty in obtaining clarification of charges or nonpayment may discourage efforts to obtain what is needed. Unfortunately, growing old does not assist one in developing new bookkeeping skills!

All health professionals understand the value of preventive examinations and would prefer that these be instituted and maintained as the basis of any health plan and particularly that they be reimbursed by Medicare. These are paramount in ensuring better and longer living. Yet, many elderly are seen only because of specific complaints and may see several health professionals who are not known to each other. As a result, there may be detrimental interactions between prescriptions drugs. Because about two-thirds of elderly people take at least one over-the-counter medication daily, there may also be harmful reactions when these are combined with prescribed medications. Many memory problems referred to psychologists result from the interaction of multiple medications.

Professionals, too, are overwhelmed by bookkeeping demands. As a result, health professionals must secure assistants whose only tasks are to complete, maintain, and follow up on multitudinous records and payments.

Emotional Problems

Older people, especially those over age seventy-five, are often at some risk of suffering from limitations in their functional ability to perform the activities of daily living. However, the severity of the illness and the common risk factors alone fail to predict the general disability of many elderly people. Multiple psychological and social factors interact with the functional capacity to influence the occurrence of, the severity of, and the general recovery from illness. Thus, the disease, the treatment of the disease, the individual's coping and adaptation, family involvement, and social networks all interact on and influence recovery.

Older individuals, like people of any other age, may experience emotional and behavioral difficulties. These problems tend, however, to be eminently treatable when access to appropriate care is available. Where this age group has the financial resources, it uses psychological services and benefits from them. Generally, half of these contacts are self-initiated. However, the mental health needs of the elderly are largely unmet and underserved. The recent inclusion of psychologists and social workers as Medicare providers may enable more individuals to gain access to mental health care.

Services for many emotional needs should be considered preventive. For example, dealing with plans for retirement, coping with loss and/or changes in one's own capacities or those of a spouse, and managing the loss of a spouse and the accompanying changes in lifestyle are all common problems that may be helped by contacts with an appropriate professional. Early management of these problems may prevent the later development of more difficulties, some emotional and some physical, that have the potential to interfere with one's quality of life.

Although many elderly remain independent, they may still feel the loss of opportunities to nurture others. They may live alone and may have no children, or their children may be far away. There is sufficient evidence to suggest that loneliness, lack of social support, isolation, alienation, and the inability to negotiate the challenges of aging and to maximize the preservation of a sense of self are often expressed in exaggerated physical symptomatology and may cause the recurrence of an old illness or the development of a series of new complaints.

Many elderly are in a chronic disease state rather than in an acute one and have problems that can be managed and mitigated even if not cured. Continuous management and oversight may be needed to raise the quality of an older person's life to standards of comfortable and productive living. Thus, care functions need to be elevated to the same valued social, political, and financial status as cure functions. Social and psychological supports can maximize adaptation to a variety of situations and can enhance coping, self-esteem, and self-control.

Where there is increased dependency, because of either decreasing abilities or illness, all family members—a spouse who may also be elderly and children who frequently are middle-aged or even "senior citizens" themselves, as well as the patient—feel the stress imposed by the new demands.

Elderly people may be less attuned to the value of psychological counseling than younger people. They may equate talking to a counselor as a weakness and sometimes feel they are "crazy" if they cannot manage the course their lives have taken. Therefore, there is a tendency to want the consultant to deal with factual problems to begin with; that is, to help find resources and to plan in concrete ways.

Sometimes, medical personnel, particularly physicians

whom the elderly have known for a long time, may be the recipients of confidences, fears, angers, and sorrows. Some are understanding; others, untrained in how to deal with psychological concerns and themselves disturbed by the feelings called up by these problems, may offer false reassurances or cliché advice or may turn aside from these concerns, even neglecting them. In these cases, patients and their families, who may be chiding themselves for being weak, become quiet and are not helped with their problems.

However, skilled professionals of all disciplines are increasingly recognizing the importance of the emotions and the role they play in the maintenance of good health and quality of life. As a result, these professionals pay attention to emotional stress and needs and accept their own abilities and limitations. Then, they are able to suggest appropriate referrals to deal with the problems that are being raised. Some of these referrals may be for psychological help; some may be to those who are skilled in management and the negotiation of the systems that offer the needed physical, economic, or emotional supports.

Professionals who are skilled in counseling the elderly recognize the pressure of external circumstances and the frequent depth of despair about various losses even if these cannot be easily put into words. As a result, they always proceed slowly, working at the pace of the patient and recognizing the impact of concrete needs and external circumstances. Attention to first things first permits the relaxation that enables better coping and therefore better living. It also assists in the prevention of various disabilities.

Physical Illness

Illness can be very frightening to the older person, who may worry about what will come next. An understanding of what the problems are and being helped to help oneself can ease this fear. It is essential to the patient that the treatment problem and plan be carefully explained, that is, what is being done or needs to be done, why, and what the possible outcomes are.

Courteous, respectful treatment helps the patient to maintain dignity and to feel more in control. Calling the elderly person by his or her first name (as may happen more frequently to women than to men) may not be perceived as being "friendly"; instead, the reaction may be a feeling of losing one's dignity and status. One elderly woman noted that she had grown up in a period when the older person was always treated with respect and always called by his or her surname and title "Now," she noted ruefully, "I am one of the elderly. We are no longer respected. Instead, we are reduced to the status of incompetents and are patronized by those who are young and healthy."

Long periods of sitting in the reception room, waiting to be seen, increase the tension that inevitably arises when one does not feel well. Sometimes, the health personnel rush in and rush out, and it is difficult to get someone to listen to one's needs. All people prefer to see helpers who are not in a rush and who will talk with them and answer their questions.

If special health needs arise, it is essential to know what services are available and helpful to have someone besides the patient and/or the family assist in making the necessary arrangements. For example there may be a need for home health aides, or special equipment or arrangement of the home. Frequently, the illness may create additional economic, physical, and/or emotional stress for the patient and the family. Help in negotiating systems and managing change may often be needed.

For example, a ninety-five-year-old man was being cared for at home by his younger wife; she was eighty years old. Even though he was seriously ill, she had no help. The problem in this case was not the failure of her physician to recognize what was needed, but her refusal to let anyone help her. To some extent, her fear was the cost and the possibility that her money would not last, so that there would be nothing left for her or anything to leave for her children. Therefore, she depended on some neighbors to assist her with her shopping. But the physical care that her husband needed was taxing her strength. In this case, some intervention was needed to work with her emotional problems and her fears and wishes about the future.

Family stress and dysfunction often occur during caregiving for impaired aged relatives, particularly when there are extensive needs for physical and/or nursing care because of incontinence, physical immobility, and mental or emotional disturbance. Extended nursing assistance is rarely available to most families because of the financial cost and, and what is provided by most health plans for care is limited. As a result, the demands on the "healthy" family members may be overwhelming. Services that compensate for functional impairments tend to be labor-intensive and expensive, and receiving such services requires many social and psychological adjustments for older people and their families. In all cases, there is great stress because of the physical and emotional demands on the caregivers.

Despite the difficult job, most family caregivers have little knowledge of what is needed and often do not have the necessary skills. Feelings of guilt, shame, and even anger may result from feelings of inadequacy; all of this may produce bad decisions and even neglect and abuse. Inadequate coping skills may also lead to feelings of depression and a reduced caregiving capacity.

Family Support

The care of choice is always the home and the family. Though caregiving activities vary widely according to the needs of the older person, the emotional support provided is one of the most important and universal caregiving task. Being in one's own home, having one's family caring for one, is always preferred over institutional care.

Yet, the care of the older person is usually provided by a spouse and, secondly, by an adult daughter and makes great demands on all. In addition, social and demographic trends, such as the disproportionate growth of the very old, decreasing nuclear family size, the geographic dispersal of families, and the increasing labor force participation of women, raise serious concerns about the family's caregiving capabilities in the future and the effects on the whole family. In addition, the capacity of economically poor families to care for their elderly is apparently extensive, and growing poverty among today's young population does not portend well for intergenerational exchanges in the future.

For example, in one family, a woman who was suffering from a malignant brain tumor was being cared for at home, where she lived with her spouse. Though she was in a home hospice that provided a variety of services, only ten hours of home health aid were paid for. The husband attempted to provide the other care, but as his wife was incapable of doing anything herself, the tasks he had were overwhelming. He called on his son and daughter and felt abandoned when they could not meet all the demands of the situation. The daughter was employed and had her own home, including school-aged children to care for; the son lived some distance away and could be of help only on weekends. The family income was not sufficient to pay for extra help; it was too much to qualify the family for Medicaid. This emergency taxed the entire family and affected its emotional climate: The father, feeling overwhelmed, considered his children selfish; the children, who were all juggling many responsibilities, felt angry and guilty at the same time. None of this was helpful to either the patient or her caretakers.

There are other situations in which family support is not helpful to the patient or to the family. Sometimes, excessive family attention leads to greater disability and the failure to return to normal activities, because family members either do too much for the patient or verbally discourage activity even though this discouragement is inappropriate. In a small percent of cases, there is even abuse of the elderly, most predominantly by spouses who feel overwhelmed.

At present, the few formal services that are available may not ease the family's burden and stress. There is a need not only for more services but for better evaluations of what is needed, what is being provided, and how. It is generally recognized that formal care cannot substitute for family care, but appropriate support of the family can enhance and enable the family's efforts. Knowledge of the adaptation of the older family to situations involving caregiving is still in the formative stage. Increased help, for both patient and family caregivers, is needed in finding ways of adapting to the specific illness and, sometimes, to the long-term implications of increased disability. Family caregivers may need specific training, which may be provided by a variety of professionals, most usually social workers and nurses. However, this is an area where greater interdisciplinary cooperation is useful.

Community-based programs funded by Medicaid waivers, Older Americans Act funds, and/or special state programs provide some long-term-care services, including home care, chore services, adult day care, home-delivered meals, and transportation. All these can assist in maintaining a reasonable home lifestyle and in preserving the dignity of the older person. The professional concerns are to acquaint the families with these services and to help obtain them. Unfortunately, as illustrated by the previous case vignette, we are still at the point where some needed services are not available or adequate for many who need them.

Care Outside the Home

Care outside the home is usually provided on an acute basis in the hospital, or chronic care is provided in a nursing home or similar institution.

Hospitalization disrupts life and heightens fears of loss of physical health and the concomitant increased dependency. Therefore, anxiety, depression, and denial are not uncommon and add additional stress to an already stressful situation. This added stress sometimes increases the risk that the frail elderly will become confused or disoriented and less able to manage the home health care necessitated by the illness. It may compromise the patient's capacity to comply with medical recommendations and may increase the likelihood of repeat hospitalizations.

Too frequently, because of cutbacks and budgetary constraints, the services that are professionally prescribed are not in sufficient supply. For example, an eighty-year-old man was hospitalized because of a series of seizures. It took much testing to determine that the cause was a new and undiagnosed diabetic problem. The patient's history included a distinguished career as a engineer, many intellectual pursuits, and a high-level verbal capacity. Nevertheless, the hospital staff spoke simply and loudly to him as one does to someone who cannot be expected to understand. His son reported that, once, when they were having difficulty helping him into his pajamas, he remarked, "This is turning into quite an undertaking" and with a sly grin added, "That's a bad choice of words." This comment not only was indicative of his capable thought process and verbal ability but was also a roundabout communication of his fear that he was dying.

In another case, a patient's condition made walking difficult for him. The physician had prescribed frequent assistance in walking in order to maintain and improve the patient's functioning; however, the shortage of nursing help made it impossible for the patient to be assisted in walking more than once a day.

Frequently, limited hospital visiting hours may not be in the best interest of the older patient, who may be fearful and lonely without family support. In such cases, consultation with the physician, the social service, and the nursing staff can clear the way for the additional support that the presence of family members may provide.

Services are needed in making the transition from the hospital to either the home or other facilities. there is a trend toward shorter acute-care hospital stays and discharges for brief recuperative stays in nursing homes if necessary. Unfortunately, many acute-care hospitals are now incapable of providing the psychotherapeutic services and psychosocial supports to patients and families that would ensure an easy transition back to the community, nor do they provide the social and psychological services, including a coordination of social, medical, and psychological supports, needed to sustain successful adaptation of the patient and family.

Undue stress caused by the hospitalization itself and inadequate assistance may increase the risk of a frail older person's becoming confused and disoriented and less able to manage the home health care that may be necessitated by the illness. This inability will compromise the capacity to comply with medical recommendations and will increase the likelihood of repeat hospitalizations.

The Common Interests of the Consumer and the Provider

For the most part, the interests of the personnel providing health services and the patients who need and use these services coincide. Both are interested in the best of services, tailored to individual needs, focused on prevention, and geared to enhancing and improving the patient's quality of life. Providers of health services have an investment in the health and the progress of the people they serve. Unfortunately, both consumer and provider suffer the effects of stringent economic measures and bureaucratic demands. There are, however, differences in some areas.

Ethical Issues

Access to Health Care

A series of problems are of ethical concern to practitioners. For example, rationing of health care is being discussed in many health and government bodies because of the high cost of current medical technology. For whom should expensive services be used: those who can pay the costs? All who need them? Those with the best chance of an improved life? These are more than "economic" issues. They concern the ethical issues of health care and the moral imperatives of a society.

The largest issue is the problem of health care of the near-poor, the impoverished, the homeless, the handicapped, those who are institutionalized, the homebound, and many living in rural areas. For all of these groups, the present services are inadequate; for some, they do not exist at all.

Issues Surrounding Living and Dying

Increasingly, there is a consideration of personal wishes about the right to live or die and/or about the use of extreme measures to prolong life. This consideration is evident in the increased use and legalization of living wills. Statistics show that for 50 percent of people, the wish of the dying person during the last two weeks of life is to be more comfortable. The question of life and death poses ethical and value questions to professionals. Many physicians believe that their job is to take care of the patient and not make decisions about life or death. For example, one physician noted that we cannot regulate life or death. His own mother, at age ninety-two, was in a coma, and the prognosis was that she would live only one to two weeks longer. Heroics were unwanted, and the "tubes" were removed; four days later, she was fine.

Recommendations Concerning Improved Care

The recommendations concerning improved health care for the elderly focus on prevention to enable longer and healthier living, an improved quality of life, and the development and improvement of health services to foster these. These recommendations serve both the provider and the consumer.

Prevention

1. Emphasis should be put on the quality of life rather than on technological advancements only. A positive developmental approach to the aging process needs to be stressed, as opposed to stressing decline.

2. If one is to take seriously the issues of health promotion and prevention, improvement is needed in diagnostic schemes and categorizations to provide services for individuals experiencing the various normal aspects of aging, such as psychosocial stressors. The present dearth of psychotherapeutic services for the elderly needs to be addressed.

3. There is a need to develop a motivation in society and in the individual to focus on the prevention and early control of disability in all age groups and to control and possibly prevent disability and premature disability in an early phases of and

illness. Changes in Medicare policies are necessary to permit payment for preventive checkups.

4. The elderly patient needs to be empowered as much as possible. Giving the elderly more sense of control will increase their morale and reduce their morbidity. Peer support is a strong health factor that tends to be present in group living arrangements and in retirement communities, particularly those with built-in health services. Educational programs and specific strategies should be tailored to enable an increase in quality of life and activeness, and access to these programs should be ensured for the elderly, who may not know about or have easily available the many opportunities that already exist, such as foster grandparents programs and programs in the arts, in business consultation, and in peer counseling, all of which increase the fullness of life. In addition, economic and social needs may be met through programs of matching roommates, shared housing, reverse mortgages, and living insurance benefits.

Access to Care

1. Effective practice with older people requires that the location of health services be truly accessible and available, such as in mobile dental clinics, Senior centers, and storefront offices, even though these may not provide the most desired resources and ambience. Senior-citizen discount programs may increase the use of dental services. In addition, the use of portable dental equipment may make available appropriate dental care for those in institutions or for those who are home-bound.

2. Because visual acuity is essential in maintaining independence, access to the latest equipment and techniques in this field should be available. There needs to be careful monitoring of changing visual needs and conditions as a result of polypharmacology. Prescription and provision (with appropriate training in use and application) of telescopic spectacles, closed-circuit Visual-Tek Type instrumentation for reading and writing, and/or perhaps a magnifier (for orthopedically involved individuals and for sewing, woodworking, painting, and other hob-

bies) can assist the elderly to maintain their autonomy, dignity, and communication with others.

3. Changes in Medicare policies to permit payment for dental and optometric care would improve access availability.

4. Access to optimal care should be available to all people, regardless of their income. This availability will require reform at all government levels to produce coordinated rather than disparate policies.

Professional Tasks

1. The first task for all of the health professions is to develop and increase their knowledge and expertise in working with people who are in the later years of life. There needs to be more understanding of and ability to help people with both retirement decisions and the adjustment to retirement, as well as with the various crises that are common occurrences during the older years.

2. Because of the burgeoning costs of health care, new concepts in health care practice in terms of facilities, diagnosis, and treatment are imperative.

3. The educational training in all professions needs updating to include essential information about and methods of helping the older person. Because of the growing need, specialities in gerontology should be considered in all of the professions. Common educational material could also stimulate an exchange of knowledge and reduce territorial attitudes and behavior.

4. A sophisticated electronically controlled information base could be used more adequately and efficiently if the data are collected from primary records. This process could help to develop a broad, reliable data base for studying trends and health issues in relationship to the elderly. Centralization of medical information about elderly patients could prevent duplication and conflicting medication prescription.

5. An aging family structure presents a compelling challenge to the helping professions. There is a need for services to engage in a systems approach that views the family as a dynamic whole and encompasses case management as well as clinical

interventions. In addition, there is a need to consider the whole patient, not only the "sick" part.

6. Effective practice with older people requires interdisciplinary collaboration so that they can be assisted appropriately with the prevention and treatment of problems in relation to their physical health and their economic and social needs. Interprofessional cooperation is a must in the proper care and understanding of the geriatric patient. There is a need for teams that work together to provide care and to prevent duplication of effort and of diagnostic tests and resultant costs. The reality of limited health-care dollars requires all professions to think together in terms of priorities as well as to evaluate together how effectively they are using the existing resources.

7. The same vigor and systematic attention needs to be paid to the later years of the life cycle as to the formative ones.

Most important of all, the effective provision of care to older people requires that we confront the power of ageism in our society, our lives, our professions, and ourselves.

Participants in Health Forum on the Aging*

Dentistry

Walter Cohen, D.D.S., President, Medical College of Pennsylvania

Gary Goldstein, D.D.S., Professor and Director of Research, Department of Prosthodontics, New York University College of Dentistry

Saul Kamen, D.D.S., Professor of Dental Health, School of Dental Medicine, State University of New York at Stony Brook

Lawrence Kerr, D.D.S., Fellow, Institute of Medicine and Past President, American Dental Association

Abraham Kobren, D.D.S., Private practice in dentistry

Peter Andrew Neff, D.D.S., Private practice in dentistry

George Zurkow, D.D.S., Clinical Professor of Endodontics, School of Dental Medicine, University of Pennsylvania

*This forum took place in Washington, DC during April 1990.

Medicine

Morris F. Collen, M.D., Consultant and Director Emeritus, Division of Research, Kaiser Permanente Medical Care Program

William R. Felts, M.D., Professor of Medicine, George Washington University

Morris Kerstein, M.D., Deissler Professor and Chair, Department of Surgery, Hahnemann University School of Medicine

Perry A. Lambird, M.D., Clinical Professor of Pathology, University of Oklahoma

Thomas Langfitt, M.D., President, Pew Charitable Trust, Washington, DC

Stanley Lesse, M.D., Faculty of Neurology, College of Physicians and Surgeons, Columbia University

Arnold M. Ludwig, M.D., Professor of Psychiatry, University of Kentucky School of Medicine

Richard Mayeux, M.D., Professor of Neurology and Psychology, College of Physicians and Surgeons, Columbia University

Jerald R. Schenken, M.D., Professor of Clinical Pathology, University of Nebraska

William Spencer, M.D., Emeritus Professor of Rehabilitation Medicine, Baylor College of Medicine

Nursing

Barbara Christman Adair, M.S.N., R.N., Associate Dean for Academic Programs, Vanderbilt University School of Nursing

Nancy L. Bohnet, M.N., R.N., President and CEO, Home Health Services

Rachel Z. Booth, Ph.D., R.N., Dean and Professor, University of Alabama School of Nursing

Luther Christman, Ph.D., Dean Emeritus, College of Nursing, Rush University

Linda R. Cronenwett, Ph.D., R.N., Director, Nursing Research, Dartmouth-Hitchcock Medical Center

Harvey Day, Ph.D., R.N., President, H. M. Day & Associates, Management Consulting Firm in Health Care Organizations

Joann M. Eland, Ph.D., R.N., Associate Professor of Nursing, University of Iowa

Patricia Hess, Ph.D., R.N., Professor of Nursing, San Francisco State University

L. Colette Jones, Ph.D., R.N., Professor and Associate Dean for Graduate Programs, College of Nursing, University of Nebraska

Sandra MacKay, Ph.D., R.N., Professor of Nursing, San Francisco State University

Gail A. Mallory, Ph.D., R.N., Associate Professor, Waynesburg College; home health nurse

Cathleen Michaels, Ph.D., R.N., Practitioner, St. Mary's Hospital/Health Center, Tucson, Arizona

James C. Pace, D.S.N., R.N., Assistant Professor, Vanderbilt University School of Nursing

Linda Phillips, Ph.D., R.N., Professor, College of Nursing, University of Arizona

Elizabeth Pugh, Ph.D., R.N., Associate Professor of Nursing, Pennsylvania State University

Kathryn Stewart-Hegedus, D.N.Sc., Assistant Professor, School of Nursing, University of Connecticut

Elvira Szigeti, Ph.D., R.N., College of Nursing, University of North Dakota

Mary Katherine Wakefield, Ph.D., R.N., Administrative Assistant to Senator Quentin Burdick

Joan E. Watson, Ph.D., R.N., Director, Nursing Administration and Nursing Education Graduate Programs, University of Pittsburgh

Thelma J. Wells, Ph.D., R.N., Professor, University of Rochester School of Nursing

David D. Williams, Ph.D., R.N., Pediatric Nurse Practitioner, College of Nursing, University of Florida

Joyce Yasko, Ph.D., R.N., Professor and Program Director, Graduate Programs in Medical, Surgical Nursing, University of Pittsburgh

Optometry

J. Davis Armistead, O.D., Private practice, Lubbock, Texas
Carl W. Childress, O.D., Private practice, Longview, Texas
Robert K. Graham, O.D., Private practice, Carlsbad, California
Robert M. Greenburg, O.D., Fellow, College of Optometrists in Vision Development
John Howlette, O.D., D.O.S., Private practice, Richmond, Virginia
William M. Ludlam, O.D., Professor, College of Optometry, Pacific University
John D. Robinson, O.D., President, National Board of Examiners in Optometry
R. Lewis Scott, O.D., Private practice, Hartford City, Indiana
W. David Sullins, Jr., O.D., D.O.S., Immediate Past President and Chair, Board of Trustees, American Optometric Association
Stanley Yamane, O.D., Vice President for Professional Relations, Vistakon

Osteopathic Medicine

Keith O. Aldridge, D.O., Trustee, American Osteopathic College of Preventive Medicine, Butler, Alabama
Stephen D. Blood, D.O., F.A.A.A.O., F.A.C.G.P., Osteopathic family physician, Alexandria, Virginia
Eileen L. DiGiovanna, D.O., Private practice, Bay Shore, New York
Joseph A. DiGiovanna, D.O., Private practice, Bay Shore, New York
Mary Elizabeth Hitchcock, D.O., Private practice, New York, New York
Howard M. Levine, D.O., Private practice, Bayonne, New Jersey
J. Jerry Rodos, D.O., Private practice, Chicago, Illinois
J. Brendan Wynne, D.O., Professor of Orthopedic Surgery, Philadelphia College of Osteopathic Medicine, Philadelphia, Pennsylvania

LeRoy E. Young, R.Ph., D.O., F.A.O.C.P., Specialist in occupational medicine

Podiatric Medicine

Charles R. Brantingham, D.P.M., Clinical Assistant Professor of Medicine, University of Southern California School of Medicine

William L. Goldfarb, D.P.M., Private practice in podiatric medicine and surgery, Bristol, Pennsylvania

Geoffrey M. Habershaw, D.P.M., Chief, Division of Podiatry, New England Deaconness Hospital, Boston, Massachusetts

Arthur E. Helfand, D.P.M., Professor and Chair, Department of Community Health and Aging, College of Podiatric Medicine, Philadelphia, Pennsylvania

Harry F. Hlavac, D.P.M., Professor of Biomechanics, California College of Podiatric Medicine

Raymond K. Locke, D.P.M., Clinical Professor, California College of Podiatric Medicine, University of Southern California at Los Angeles

Elizabeth H. Roberts, D.P.M., Professor Emerita, New York College of Podiatric Medicine

Harold D. Schoenhaus, D.P.M., Chief of Podiatric Surgery, Graduate Hospital of Philadelphia

Kove Schwartz, D.P.M., Past President, American Podiatric Medical Association

Psychology

Jules Barron, Ph.D., Private practice in clinical psychology, Westwood, New Jersey

Nina Barron, Ph.D., Private practice in clinical psychology, Westwood, New Jersey

Toni Bernay, Ph.D., Private practice in psychology, Beverly Hills, California

Patricia M. Bricklin, Ph.D., Professor, Institute for Graduate Clinical Psychology, Widener University

Matilda B. Canter, Ph.D., Clinical and consulting psychologist, Phoenix, Arizona

Dorothy W. Cantor, Psy.D., Private practice in psychology, Westfield, New Jersey

Nicholas A. Cummings, Ph.D., Chair and CEO, American Biodyne, Inc., and Past President, American Psychological Association

Patrick De Leon, Ph.D., Administrative assistant to U.S. Senator D. K. Inouye

Ronald Fox, Ph.D., Dean, School of Professional Psychology, Wright State University

Herbert Freudenberger, Ph.D., Private practice in psychoanalysis, New York, New York

Robert Harper, Ph.D., Private practice in clinical psychology, Washington, DC

Molly Harrower, Ph.D., Professor Emerita, University of Florida

Wilbur E. Morley, Ph.D., Private practice, Los Angeles, California

Bernard Riess, Ph.D., Training Analyst and Senior Supervisor, Postgraduate Center for Mental Health, New York, New York

Hirsch Lazaar Silverman, Ph.D., Private practice in clinical and forensic psychological services, West Orange, New Jersey

Faith Tanney, Ph.D., Private practice in psychology, Washington, DC

Gary R. VandenBos, Ph.D., American Psychological Association, Washington, DC

Bryant L. Welch, Ph.D., Executive Director of Practice Directorate, American Psychological Association

Social Work

Barbara Berkman, D.S.W., Director of Research, Social Service Department, Massachusetts General Hospital, and Associate Director, Geriatric Education Center, Harvard University School of Medicine

Morris Black, M.S.S., Director of Community Services, Jewish Board of Family and Children's Services, New York, New York

Phyllis Caroff, D.S.W., Professor Emerita, Hunter College School of Social Work, City University of New York, New York, New York

Shirley S. Carroll, M.S.W., Clinical Social Worker, Central Psychiatric Clinic, Cleveland, Ohio

Rose Dobrof, D.S.W., Director, Brookdale Center on Aging, and Co-Director, Hunter/Mt. Sinai Geriatric Education Center

Ann Farwell, M.S.S.W., Adjunct Associate Professor, Smith College School for Social Work

Jerome M. Goldsmith, Ed.D., Executive Director, Jewish Board of Family and Children's Services, New York, New York

Helen Herring, M.S.W., Private practice in clinical social work, Lexington, Kentucky

Judith M. Holm, M.S.W., Private practice in clinical social work, Cleveland, Ohio

Rosalie A. Kane, D.S.W., Professor, School of Social Work and School of Public Health, University of Minnesota

Arnold Levin, Ph.D., President, Institute for Clinical Social Work, Chicago, Illinois

Elizabeth Lewis, Ph.D., Professor, Department of Social Service, Cleveland State University

Florence Lieberman, D.S.W., Professor Emerita, Hunter College School of Social Work, City University of New York, New York, New York

Patricia T. Nitzburg, M.S.W., Director, Jewish Board of Family and Children's Services, New York, New York

Tikvah Portnoi, M.S.W., Private practice in clinical social work, Newton Center, Massachusetts

Mildred Reynolds, Ed.D., Pastoral and clinical social worker, Kensington, Maryland

Edna F. Roth, Ph.D., Professor Emerita, School of Social Work, Virginia Commonwealth University, Richmond, Virginia

Betty Jean Synar, M.S.W., Chief Social Worker, Dallas Child Guidance Clinic, Dallas, Texas

Veterinary Medicine

Leo K. Bustad, D.V.M., Professor and Dean Emeritus, College of Veterinary Medicine, Pullman, Washington, and Director, People–Pet Partnership Program

William D. Carlson, D.V.M., President Emeritus, University of Wyoming

D. K. Detweiler, D.V.M., Professor of Physiology Emeritus, University of Pennsylvania School of Veterinary Medicine

David M. Drennan, D.V.M., Private practice, pet animal veterinarian, Tallmadge, Ohio

Billy E. Hooper, D.V.M., Executive Director, Association of American Veterinary Medical Colleges

William J. Kay, D.V.M., Chief of Staff, Animal Medical Center, New York, New York

Richard M. McCapes, D.V.M., Chair, Department of Epidemiology and Preventive Medicine, School of Veterinary Medicine, University of California

John B. McCarthy, D.V.M., Senior Program Specialist, American Veterinary Medical Association

Benny Osburn, D.V.M., Associate Dean, Research and Graduate Education, School of Veterinary Medicine, Davis, California

Benjamin S. Pomeroy, D.V.M., Professor of Veterinary Microbiology, Department of Veterinary Pathobiology, College of Veterinary Medicine, University of Minnesota

Edward Rhode, D.V.M., Dean, School of Veterinary Medicine, University of California

Bud Tennant, D.V.M., James Low Professor of Comparative Medicine, Cornell University

Index